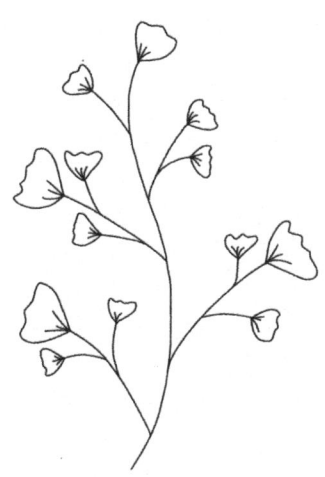

Home Herbalism for Beginners
Working with Healing Plants at Home

Shannon Reed

© 2026 Shannon Reed

Published by Field Studies Sanctuary LLC

Helena, Montana

ISBN: 978-1-969366-00-0

All rights reserved.

A LEARNING COMPANION
FOR HOME HERBALISM

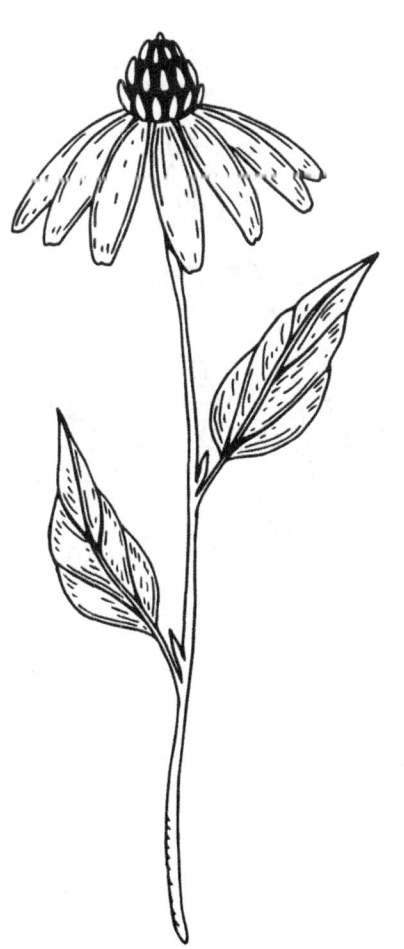

This collection was created as part of the Field Studies Sanctuary Apothecary & Learning Kitchen, a space where plant medicine is approached with curiosity, respect, and a commitment to real study. It serves as both a teaching tool and a practical home resource while offering foundational learning alongside clear guidance when support is needed.

The remedies and plant profiles gathered here reflect those most often used in everyday life. They were chosen for their safety, accessibility, and their ability to illustrate core patterns of herbalism:

- **calming the nervous system**
- **settling digestion**
- **supporting immunity**
- **easing the breath**
- **nourishing the body through periods of change and strain**

These plants form the groundwork from which deeper herbal knowledge grows.

This companion is meant to be opened often, used freely, and returned to over time. The language is intentionally simple, allowing beginners to move with confidence while offering experienced learners a steady return to the essentials. It is also designed to evolve - a working document that can expand as your apothecary deepens and your understanding widens.

Whether you are caring for yourself, your household, or your community, may this companion grow into both a useful reference and a meaningful record - one that supports your needs now while offering a clear, welcoming foundation for those who will learn from you in the years ahead.

Home Herbalism for Beginners

table of contents

- i   A Note of Gratitude
- ii   On Use & Responsibility
- iii   How to Work with This Companion

- 01   Section One · Nerves & Sleep
- 15   Section Two · Digestion & Gut Support
- 30   Section Three · Respiratory & Immune Support
- 52   Section Four · Inflammation & Pain Support
- 69   Section Five · Hormone & Cyclical Support
- 88   Section Six · Energy, Vitality, & Mood
- 100   Section Seven · Circulation & Heart Support
- 115   Section Eight · Skin & Lymph Detox

- 130   Working with the Preparations
- 142   Foundational Home Remedies
- 151   Plant Reference by Support Area
- 152   Honoring Indigenous Lineages of Plant Knowledge
- 153   Sustainable Practices, Ethical Sourcing & Foraging

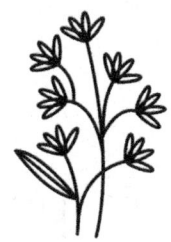

a note of gratitude

This work begins with gratitude for Mama Nature, whose generosity shapes every remedy in these pages. The plants at the center of this companion are not commodities but living teachers who offering nourishment, comfort, and guidance to anyone willing to slow down and listen. Their gifts have supported human life since the beginning, and they continue to do so even as the pace of our world pulls many of us far from that relationship.

We also honor the wisdom keepers, ancestors, and cultures who have tended these teachings across generations. The knowledge shared here does not exist in isolation. It is part of a long lineage of Indigenous practices, traditional remedies, and earth-based ways of knowing. Their stewardship is the reason we have access to this learning today, and it is our responsibility to approach these plants with respect, humility, and care.

The Field Studies Sanctuary was created with this intention in mind: to help us remember our connection to the land, to our bodies, and to one another. When we learn to work with the plants around us - and when we understand the impact our choices have on the ecosystems that sustain us - we begin to repair what has been forgotten and nurture what still thrives.

This companion is one small part of that mission. It offers an accessible place to begin, while also inviting deeper awareness of the relationships that make healing possible.

As you move through these pages, may you feel supported by the plants, grounded by the earth beneath your feet, and encouraged to participate in the quiet work of tending the world we share. -sr

on use & responsibility

The information shared in this book is offered for educational and informational purposes. It reflects traditional practices, experiential learning, and contemporary herbal understanding gathered through study, observation, and relationship with plants. These pages are intended to support curiosity, awareness, and personal exploration rather than replace professional medical care.

Plant medicine works in relationship with the body, environment, and individual history. Each person's experience will differ, and attentive listening remains essential. When working with new plants or preparations, beginning gently and observing response supports clarity and safety.

This book does not diagnose conditions, prescribe treatment, or offer medical advice. Those managing chronic illness, using prescription medications, navigating pregnancy, or working with complex health concerns are encouraged to seek guidance from a qualified healthcare practitioner or trained clinical herbalist.

Some remedies referenced here are intended for external use only or for short-term, practitioner-guided application. These are clearly noted throughout the book. Responsibility for use rests with the reader, guided by discernment, respect for the plants, and care for the body.

This work honors the long traditions of plant medicine while recognizing that modern contexts, bodies, and circumstances vary widely. May this book serve as a supportive companion, encouraging thoughtful engagement, humility, and responsibility as each reader develops their own relationship with the living world.

working with this companion

Home Herbalism for Beginners offers a steady place to meet and work with the extraordinary plants that support everyday life. It holds space for moments when the body feels unsettled, strained, or slightly out of rhythm, and it welcomes curiosity alongside need. Some readers arrive through study and interest, while others come through discomfort or a quiet inner signal asking for attention. Each path of arrival carries meaning, and each offers a doorway into learning through care, observation, and relationship.

The plants gathered in these pages support relationship with the body through presence and awareness. They work in conversation with living systems, responding to patterns that unfold over time. This book encourages returning to listening as a first step, allowing sensation, energy, and emotion to offer guidance. Attention becomes the starting place.

When opening this companion, begin by slowing the pace. Notice how the body feels physically, emotionally, and energetically. Observe patterns that repeat or sensations that ask for care. Fatigue, tension, restlessness, heaviness, heat, or depletion often speak clearly when given space. The sections of this book are organized to support this kind of noticing, offering pathways that align with common expressions of imbalance.

Some readers choose to move through the book gradually, becoming familiar with plants and preparations over time. Others reach for it in specific moments, guided by what the body expresses. Both approaches support understanding. Learning unfolds through experience as much as through reading.

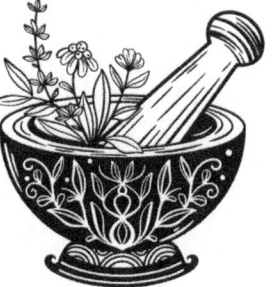

This format invites simplicity. One plant or one preparation offers enough support to begin building relationship. Consistent, gentle engagement allows clarity to develop naturally. Beginning with small amounts and observing response supports safety and awareness while strengthening trust in the process.

Preparation methods and foundational remedies appear throughout the book as points of orientation. These methods reflect practices that have supported households and communities for generations, using materials that often remain close at hand. Food, warmth, rest, movement, and touch work alongside plants, shaping conditions that support balance. Healing often emerges through patterns of care rather than single actions.

The body carries intelligence shaped by experience, environment, and history. Plant medicine supports this intelligence by addressing underlying patterns and encouraging system-wide balance. Signals that arise through discomfort or imbalance often serve as communication. Listening to these signals supports responsive care and informed choice.

People engage with health and healing through many pathways. Some feel steadied by established medical systems and professional authority. Others feel drawn toward relational, earth-based approaches that emphasize self-awareness and participation. This companion honors a wide range of choices and encourages discernment in all forms of care. Safety remains central, and professional guidance holds an important place when circumstances call for it.

Relationship with plants includes responsibility. Sustainable practices, ethical sourcing, and thoughtful foraging support both ecological health and cultural respect. When plants are gathered, restraint and gratitude shape the exchange. When plants are purchased, sourcing that honors land, labor, and lineage strengthens the integrity of the work. Care for the body and care for the Earth remain connected.

The natural world offers countless examples of intuitive care. Animals seek out specific plants, minerals, and environments when injured or strained, guided by sensation and instinct. Humans share this capacity. Relearning how to listen to the body reconnects instinct with awareness. This book serves as a bridge toward that remembering.

This companion supports quiet use. The choices made here unfold privately, shaped by individual rhythms and needs. Small, consistent shifts often create meaningful change over time. These practices require presence rather than performance.

If these pages encourage pausing when the body speaks, choosing care with intention, and approaching plants with respect and curiosity, they serve their purpose. May this companion offer steadiness during uncertainty, encouragement during exploration, and reassurance that meaningful relationship with the living world remains available. The doorway stands open. Move at a pace that feels true, and allow understanding to grow through experience.

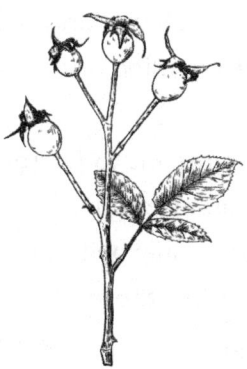

SECTION ONE

NERVES & SLEEP

This section gathers plants traditionally relied upon to support the nervous system and the rhythms of rest that allow the body to recover, adapt, and renew. These medicines address the many ways tension, fatigue, and overstimulation show up in daily life - from restless nights and busy minds to emotional strain held quietly beneath the surface.

Within these pages, each plant offers a distinct form of support. Some bring gentle reassurance, easing frayed nerves and encouraging the body to soften into rest. Others provide steady nourishment, rebuilding resilience after prolonged stress or depletion. A few act more decisively, helping release deeply held tension or restore balance when the system struggles to settle on its own. Together, they illustrate the wide range of ways plants meet the nervous system where it is and guide it toward greater ease.

The remedies featured here are among those most commonly reached for in moments of stress, sleeplessness, and emotional fatigue. They were chosen for their accessibility, familiarity, and their ability to demonstrate core principles of herbal support for the nervous system - calming, restoring, steadying, and strengthening over time. Through working with them, patterns begin to emerge that deepen understanding and build confidence.

This section is meant to be returned to often, whether for immediate support or quiet study. It invites observation, patience, and an ongoing relationship with the plants that help the body remember how to rest. May these pages offer a reliable starting place and a steady companion as you learn to listen more closely to the needs of your nervous system and the rhythms that sustain it.

ashwagandha
passionflower
chamomile
oatstraw
lemon balm
lavender
catnip
motherwort
damiana
st. john's wort
valerian
schisandra
rosemary

ASHWAGANDHA
withania somnifera

balance

HOW SHE MIGHT HELP

Periods of prolonged stress, exhaustion, and nervous system depletion often call for Ashwagandha, especially when the body feels worn down and rest arrives with difficulty.

WORKING WITH HER

Steady, regular use allows Ashwagandha to offer her fullest support. She is commonly taken as a tincture, powder, or infusion and integrates smoothly into morning or early evening routines. Benefits tend to build gradually through consistent relationship over time.

AVOID COMBINING

Greater harmony is found when Ashwagandha is used apart from other strong, energizing adaptogens such as rhodiola or eleuthero taken at the same time. Care also serves when combining with strong warming herbs taken in high doses, including ginger, cayenne, cinnamon, or garlic, particularly when the body already feels overstimulated.

IMPORTANT NOTES

During pregnancy, Ashwagandha is set aside. Thoughtful use also supports those with hyperthyroidism, and careful attention is encouraged when combined with sedative or thyroid medications. Her greatest benefit emerges through steady, long-term support, beginning with a low dose and attentive observation of the body's response.

COMMON PREPARATIONS*

Tea (decoction)
Tincture
Powder
Capsule
Ghee or honey-based paste

*See the Preparation Guide in the back of this book

WORKS WELL WITH

oatstraw
lemon balm
holy basil (tulsi)
reishi mushroom
licorice root

Long valued in traditional systems for restoring balance after depletion, Ashwagandha reminds the body how to settle and recover.

PASSIONFLOWER
passiflora incarnata

calm

HOW SHE MIGHT HELP
When the nervous system feels overactive and the mind struggles to settle, Passionflower offers support during moments of restlessness, anxious tension, and difficulty easing into sleep.

WORKING WITH HER
Gentle consistency allows Passionflower to express her calming nature most fully. She is commonly taken as a tincture or infusion and fits naturally into evening or pre-bed routines. With ongoing use, the nervous system often finds greater ease in releasing excess stimulation.

AVOID COMBINING
Greater balance is supported when Passionflower is used apart from other strong sedative herbs taken in high doses at the same time. Thoughtful attention also serves when combining with pharmaceutical sedatives, as their effects may feel intensified together.

IMPORTANT NOTES
Sensitivity to sedative effects invites a mindful approach when working with Passionflower. Careful attention is encouraged for those taking sedative medications, and beginning with a low dose supports clarity in observing the body's response as the relationship develops.

COMMON PREPARATIONS*

Tea (infusion)
Tincture
Glycerite

*See the Preparation Guide in the back of this book

WORKS WELL WITH

lemon balm
skullcap
oatstraw
chamomile
lavender

Known for her steadying influence on an overactive mind, Passionflower helps guide the body toward calm and restorative rest.

CHAMOMILE
matricaria chamomilla

soften

HOW SHE MIGHT HELP
Gentle nervous tension, digestive unease linked to stress, and difficulty winding down often invite the support of Chamomile, especially when rest feels close yet elusive.

WORKING WITH HER
Soft, regular contact allows Chamomile's calming qualities to unfold with ease. She is most often taken as an infusion and fits naturally into evening rituals or moments that call for grounding and comfort. With consistent use, the nervous system frequently settles alongside the body.

AVOID COMBINING
Greater ease is supported when Chamomile is used apart from other strong sedative herbs taken in high doses at the same time. Attentive use also serves those with known sensitivities to plants in the daisy family.

IMPORTANT NOTES
Sensitivity to mild sedative effects invites a mindful approach when working with Chamomile. Thoughtful attention supports those with plant allergies, and beginning gently allows the body's response to guide the relationship.

COMMON PREPARATIONS*

Tea (infusion)
Compress or poultice
Steam

*See the Preparation Guide in the back of this book

WORKS WELL WITH

lemon balm
lavender
oatstraw
passionflower
rose

Often turned to for comfort and quiet reassurance, Chamomile supports the nervous system in softening its grip and settling into rest.

OATSTRAW
avena sativa

HOW SHE MIGHT HELP
Periods of nervous exhaustion, emotional depletion, and long-term stress often draw attention to Oatstraw, especially when the system feels worn thin and in need of steady nourishment.

WORKING WITH HER
Slow, consistent relationship allows Oatstraw to offer her deepest support. She is most often taken as a long infusion and weaves easily into daily routines focused on rebuilding and restoration. Over time, her mineral-rich presence supports resilience within the nervous system.

AVOID COMBINING
Oatstraw integrates smoothly alongside many gentle nervine and nourishing herbs and is generally easy to combine within broader formulations. Attentive use supports those with sensitivities to oats, particularly where sourcing and preparation matter.

IMPORTANT NOTES
Long-term use suits Oatstraw's nourishing nature and supports gradual replenishment rather than immediate effect. Careful sourcing benefits those with gluten sensitivity, as only the straw of the oat plant is used. Gentle consistency allows her benefits to unfold steadily.

---

ease

COMMON PREPARATIONS*

Tea
(long infusion or overnight infusion)
Tincture
Herbal vinegar
Bath soak or compress

*See the Preparation Guide in the back of this book

WORKS WELL WITH

lemon balm
passionflower
chamomile
nettle
milky oats

Valued for her deeply restorative qualities, Oatstraw offers steady nourishment that helps the nervous system regain strength and ease.

LEMON BALM
melissa officinalis

soothe

HOW SHE MIGHT HELP
Gentle anxiety, nervous tension, and restlessness shaped by an overactive mind often soften in the presence of Lemon Balm, especially when the heart and nervous system feel unsettled together.

WORKING WITH HER
Regular, gentle use allows Lemon Balm's calming nature to emerge with clarity. She is most often taken as an infusion or tincture and fits easily into daily rhythms during periods of stress. Consistency supports a sense of ease within the nervous system.

AVOID COMBINING
Greater ease is often found when Lemon Balm is taken separately from other calming herbs used in high doses, giving the nervous system space to respond gradually. Attentive use also serves those working with thyroid medications.

IMPORTANT NOTES
Lemon Balm suits gentle, ongoing use and is generally well tolerated. Careful attention supports those with thyroid considerations, and beginning moderately allows the body's response to guide the relationship over time.

COMMON PREPARATIONS*

Tea (infusion, fresh or dried)
Tincture
Glycerite
Honey infusion

*See the Preparation Guide in the back of this book

WORKS WELL WITH

oatstraw
passionflower
chamomile
skullcap
rose

Known for her uplifting calm and steadying presence, Lemon Balm helps soothe the nervous system while gently lifting the spirit.

LAVENDER
lavandula angustifolia

settle

HOW SHE MIGHT HELP

Subtle nervous tension, sensory overwhelm, and difficulty settling often soften with Lavender, especially when the system feels keyed up and in need of gentle reassurance.

WORKING WITH HER

Light, consistent use allows Lavender's calming qualities to emerge without heaviness. She is commonly taken as an infusion, tincture, or aromatic preparation and fits naturally into evening routines or moments that call for quieting the senses. Regular use supports a softened nervous response.

AVOID COMBINING

Balance is supported when Lavender is used apart from other strong sedative herbs taken in high doses at the same time. Attentive spacing also serves when combining with pharmaceutical sedatives, as effects may feel more pronounced together.

IMPORTANT NOTES

Lavender is generally well tolerated and suits gentle, ongoing use. Sensitivity to aroma or taste invites a lighter hand, allowing the body's response to guide continued relationship.

COMMON PREPARATIONS*

Tea (infusion)
Tincture
Essential oil (aromatic use)
Pillow sachet or compress

*See the Preparation Guide in the back of this book

WORKS WELL WITH

lemon balm
chamomile
oatstraw
passionflower
rose

Often turned to for soothing both nerves and senses, Lavender helps the body settle into calm through quiet, steady presence.

CATNIP
nepeta cataria

rest

HOW SHE MIGHT HELP
Gentle nervous agitation, restlessness, and tension that show up alongside digestive unease often ease with Catnip, especially when the body seeks comfort and relaxation together.

WORKING WITH HER
Soft, regular use allows Catnip's calming nature to express itself clearly. She is most often taken as a warm infusion and integrates easily into evening routines or moments that call for soothing and release. Consistency supports relaxation without heaviness.

AVOID COMBINING
Catnip tends to blend smoothly with other gentle nervines and calming herbs. Attentive use supports balance when combining with stronger sedative herbs taken in high doses at the same time.

IMPORTANT NOTES
Catnip suits mild, ongoing support and is generally well tolerated. Beginning gently allows the body's response to guide continued relationship, particularly for those sensitive to sedative effects.

COMMON PREPARATIONS*

Tea (infusion)
Tincture
Bath soak or compress

*See the Preparation Guide in the back of this book

WORKS WELL WITH

chamomile
lemon balm
oatstraw
lavender
fennel

Often valued for her comforting presence, Catnip supports relaxation by gently easing the nervous system and inviting the body to rest.

MOTHERWORT
leonurus cardiaca

calm

HOW SHE MIGHT HELP
Moments of emotional turbulence, nervous tension held in the chest, and restlessness shaped by stress often call for Motherwort, especially when the heart and nerves feel entwined.

WORKING WITH HER
Steady, attentive use allows Motherwort's grounding influence to come forward. She is most often taken as a tincture or infusion and fits naturally into routines that support emotional regulation and nervous system balance. Over time, her presence encourages steadiness and ease.

AVOID COMBINING
Motherwort integrates best when used apart from other strong sedative herbs taken in high doses at the same time. Thoughtful spacing also supports harmony when combining with cardiac or sedative medications.

IMPORTANT NOTES
Motherwort is traditionally set aside during pregnancy due to her uterine influence. Careful attention also serves those working with heart-related medications, and beginning gently allows the body's response to guide continued relationship.

COMMON PREPARATIONS*

Tincture
Tea (infusion)
Glycerite
Poultice or compress

*See the Preparation Guide in the back of this book

WORKS WELL WITH

lemon balm
hawthorn
oatstraw
passionflower
rose

Long associated with steadying the heart in times of strain, Motherwort supports emotional balance by calming the nervous system and anchoring the body in presence.

DAMIANA
turnera diffusa

support   10

HOW SHE MIGHT HELP
Nervous tension shaped by fatigue, emotional flatness, or low mood often responds well to Damiana, especially when restlessness and depletion appear together.

WORKING WITH HER
Gentle, consistent use allows Damiana's balancing qualities to emerge clearly. She is most often taken as an infusion or tincture and fits easily into routines that support nervous system ease alongside restored vitality. Over time, her presence supports relaxation without dulling awareness.

AVOID COMBINING
Damiana integrates best when used apart from other strong stimulating or sedative herbs taken in high doses at the same time. Thoughtful spacing supports balance when combining with herbs or substances that strongly influence mood or energy.

IMPORTANT NOTES
Damiana suits moderate, ongoing use and is generally well tolerated. Beginning gently supports clarity in observing the body's response, particularly for those sensitive to shifts in energy or mood.

COMMON PREPARATIONS*

Tea (infusion)
Tincture
Smoking blend or aromatic preparation

*See the Preparation Guide in the back of this book

WORKS WELL WITH

oatstraw
passionflower
lemon balm
rose
cacao

Often valued for restoring ease and quiet vitality, Damiana supports the nervous system in softening while gently reawakening embodied presence.

ST. JOHN'S WORT
hypericum perforatum

steady

HOW SHE MIGHT HELP

Periods of low mood, nervous fatigue, and sensitivity to emotional or sensory overload often draw attention to St. John's Wort, especially when light and resilience feel diminished.

WORKING WITH HER

Intentional, consistent use allows St. John's Wort to express her stabilizing qualities. She is most often taken as a tincture, infused oil, or tea and fits best into routines that support steadiness over time. Regular relationship supports gradual nervous system balance.

AVOID COMBINING

Greater ease is found when St. John's Wort is used apart from pharmaceuticals that influence mood, hormones, or nervous system signaling. Careful attention also serves when combining with herbs that strongly stimulate or sedate the system.

IMPORTANT NOTES

St. John's Wort carries a strong affinity for nervous system chemistry and benefits from informed, attentive use. Increased sensitivity to sunlight may arise, and careful observation supports clarity as the body responds over time.

COMMON PREPARATIONS*

Tincture
Tea (infusion)
Infused oil (external use)

*See the Preparation Guide in the back of this book

WORKS WELL WITH

lemon balm
oatstraw
rose
lavender
skullcap

Long associated with restoring inner light and resilience, St. John's Wort supports the nervous system in regaining steadiness and emotional clarity.

VALERIAN
valeriana officinalis

unwind

HOW SHE MIGHT HELP
Persistent nervous tension, difficulty falling asleep, and overstimulation that resists gentler support often call for Valerian, especially when the system feels wired and unable to settle.

WORKING WITH HER
Measured, intentional use allows Valerian's calming influence to emerge clearly. She is most often taken as a tincture, decoction, or capsule and fits naturally into evening or nighttime routines. With consistent use, the nervous system often releases held tension more fully.

AVOID COMBINING
Balance is supported when Valerian is worked with apart from other strong sedative herbs taken in high doses at the same time. Thoughtful attention also serves when combining with pharmaceutical sedatives, as effects may feel amplified together.

IMPORTANT NOTES
Valerian carries a deep affinity for the nervous system and supports rest through gradual settling, with individual responses varying as the body acclimates to her presence over time.

COMMON PREPARATIONS*
Tincture
Tea (decoction or long infusion)
Glycerite
Capsule

Note: Valerian root is most often prepared with longer steeping or extraction methods to support full expression of her grounding qualities.

*See the Preparation Guide in the back of this book

WORKS WELL WITH
lemon balm
oatstraw
rose
lavender
skullcap

Long regarded as a guide into restorative sleep, Valerian supports the nervous system in releasing tension and rediscovering rest through gentle unwinding.

SCHISANDRA
schisandra chinensis

resilience

HOW SHE MIGHT HELP
Times of nervous fatigue, stress held deep in the system, and difficulty maintaining equilibrium often invite Schisandra, especially when resilience and focus feel diminished.

WORKING WITH HER
Steady, intentional use allows Schisandra's balancing qualities to unfold. She is commonly taken as a tincture, powder, or decoction and integrates well into daily routines that support endurance and nervous system regulation. Ongoing relationship supports clarity and adaptability over time.

AVOID COMBINING
Harmony is supported when Schisandra is used apart from other strong adaptogens taken in high doses at the same time. Thoughtful attention also serves when combining with medications that strongly influence liver metabolism or nervous system signaling.

IMPORTANT NOTES
Schisandra carries a concentrated, tonifying character and suits measured, consistent use. Beginning gently supports clear observation of the body's response, particularly for those sensitive to stimulating effects.

COMMON PREPARATIONS*

Tea (decoction)
Tincture
Powder
Honey-based preparations

*See the Preparation Guide in the back of this book

WORKS WELL WITH

oatstraw
reishi mushroom
lemon balm
rose
astragalus

Traditionally valued for strengthening resilience under stress, Schisandra supports the nervous system in maintaining balance while meeting sustained demand.

ROSEMARY
salvia rosmarinus

clarity

HOW SHE MIGHT HELP

Mental fatigue, sluggish focus, and nervous dullness often benefit from Rosemary, especially when clarity and alert calm feel difficult to sustain.

WORKING WITH HER

Intentional, moderate use allows Rosemary's enlivening qualities to support the nervous system without tipping into excess. She is most often taken as an infusion, tincture, or aromatic preparation and fits well into morning or daytime routines. Regular relationship supports mental clarity and steady engagement.

AVOID COMBINING

Greater balance is found when Rosemary is used apart from other strongly stimulating herbs taken in high doses at the same time. Thoughtful attention also serves when combining with substances or medications that markedly increase stimulation.

IMPORTANT NOTES

Rosemary carries a warming, activating nature and suits measured use. Beginning gently supports awareness of the body's response, particularly for those sensitive to stimulation or heat.

COMMON PREPARATIONS*

Tea (infusion)
Tincture
Infused oil (external use)
Aromatic preparation

*See the Preparation Guide in the back of this book

WORKS WELL WITH

lemon balm
lavender
oatstraw
sage
rose

Often turned to for sharpening awareness and lifting mental fog, Rosemary supports the nervous system in meeting the day with clarity and presence.

SECTION TWO

DIGESTION & GUT SUPPORT

Digestive health shapes how nourishment is received, how energy is sustained, and how the body responds to daily demands. The gut reflects rhythm, resilience, and adaptability, responding quickly to stress, environment, and habit. When digestion feels supported, the entire system often settles into greater balance.

The plants gathered here approach digestive care from many directions. Some awaken appetite and encourage healthy digestive flow, preparing the body to receive food with ease. Others soothe irritation, protect delicate tissues, or support the movement of stagnation that builds quietly over time. Several of these remedies illustrate the close relationship between digestion and liver function, highlighting how assimilation and elimination work together to support vitality.

Roots, seeds, leaves, and blended formulas appear throughout these pages because of their familiarity and practical value. They demonstrate foundational digestive patterns such as warming and cooling, stimulating and calming, drying and moistening. Working with them reveals how digestion responds to timing, consistency, and thoughtful preparation.

These pages invite regular return and close observation. Attention to appetite, comfort, and elimination becomes a form of listening, guided by plants that have long supported digestive resilience. May this collection offer a steady entry point into gut care and deepen understanding of the relationships that allow nourishment to be received with ease.

gentian root
plantain leaf
ginger root
fennel seeds
chicory root
triphala
dandelion root
turmeric
licorice root
act. charcoal*
bitters
marshmallow
slippery elm
peppermint

GENTIAN ROOT
gentiana lutea

awaken

HOW SHE MIGHT HELP
Sluggish digestion, low appetite, and a sense of heaviness after meals often respond to Gentian, especially when digestive fire feels diminished or slow to engage.

WORKING WITH HER
Small, intentional use allows Gentian's bitter qualities to activate digestive readiness. She is most often taken as a tincture or tea and is traditionally worked with shortly before meals. Consistent relationship supports improved appetite and digestive flow over time.

AVOID COMBINING
Gentian tends to serve best when not layered with other strong bitter herbs used in high doses at the same time. Careful attention also supports those experiencing active gastric irritation, as her stimulating nature may feel intense when tissues are already inflamed.

IMPORTANT NOTES
Gentian carries a strong bitter profile and is well suited to measured use. Beginning gently supports clarity in observing the body's response, particularly for those sensitive to digestive stimulation.

COMMON PREPARATIONS*

Tincture
Tea (decoction)
Digestive bitters

*See the Preparation Guide in the back of this book

WORKS WELL WITH

ginger root
fennel seeds
chicory root
dandelion root
peppermint

Long valued for awakening digestion through bitterness, Gentian helps the body prepare to receive nourishment with greater strength and clarity.

PLANTAIN LEAF
plantago major

soothe

HOW SHE MIGHT HELP
Irritation along the digestive tract, minor inflammation, and discomfort linked to sensitive tissues often ease with Plantain, especially when the gut benefits from soothing and protection.

WORKING WITH HER
Gentle, steady use allows Plantain's cooling and drawing qualities to come forward. She is most often taken as an infusion or tincture and fits well into routines that support tissue repair and digestive comfort. Ongoing relationship supports calm, resilient digestion.

AVOID COMBINING
Plantain integrates smoothly alongside many gentle digestive and soothing herbs. Thoughtful attention serves when combining with strong drying or stimulating remedies used in high amounts, as balance supports comfort.

IMPORTANT NOTES
Plantain is generally well tolerated and suits ongoing use. Careful sourcing supports those harvesting locally, and beginning gently allows the body's response to guide continued relationship.

COMMON PREPARATIONS*

Tea (infusion)
Tincture
Poultice or compress

*See the Preparation Guide in the back of this book

WORKS WELL WITH

marshmallow root
slippery elm
chamomile
peppermint
dandelion root

Often relied upon for its soothing and protective nature, Plantain supports digestive comfort by calming irritation and strengthening tissue resilience.

GINGER ROOT
ingiber officinale

warmth

HOW SHE MIGHT HELP
Cold digestion, sluggish movement, and discomfort marked by bloating or nausea often benefit from Ginger, especially when warmth and circulation support digestive ease.

WORKING WITH HER
Moderate, consistent use allows Ginger's warming qualities to support digestion without excess. She is most often taken as a fresh infusion, decoction, tincture, or powder and fits well into routines that encourage digestive movement and comfort. Regular relationship supports steady digestive engagement.

AVOID COMBINING
Ginger serves best when not layered heavily with other strongly heating herbs used in high amounts. Attentive use also supports those sensitive to warmth or intensity within the digestive tract.

IMPORTANT NOTES
Ginger carries a warming, activating nature and suits measured use. Beginning gently supports awareness of the body's response, particularly for those prone to heat or irritation.

COMMON PREPARATIONS*

Tea (infusion or decoction)
Fresh juice
Tincture
Powder
Poultice or compress

*See the Preparation Guide in the back of this book

WORKS WELL WITH

fennel seeds
peppermint
turmeric root
licorice root
dandelion root

Long valued for bringing warmth and movement to digestion, Ginger helps the body process nourishment with greater comfort and vitality.

FENNEL SEEDS
foeniculum vulgare

ease

HOW SHE MIGHT HELP
Gas, cramping, and digestive discomfort marked by tension or stagnation often soften with Fennel, especially when digestion benefits from gentle movement and release.

WORKING WITH HER
Gentle, regular use allows Fennel's carminative qualities to support digestive comfort. She is most often taken as a warm infusion, lightly crushed before steeping, and fits well into routines that follow meals or moments of digestive strain. Consistency supports ease and settling.

AVOID COMBINING
Fennel blends smoothly with many digestive herbs and tends to feel balanced on her own. Attentive use supports comfort when combining with stronger stimulating remedies used in high amounts.

IMPORTANT NOTES
Fennel is generally well tolerated and suits mild, ongoing support. Beginning gently supports clear observation of the body's response, particularly for those sensitive to aromatic herbs.

COMMON PREPARATIONS*

Tea
(infusion, lightly crushed seeds)
Tincture
Powder
Chewed seeds

*See the Preparation Guide in the back of this book

WORKS WELL WITH

ginger root
peppermint
chamomile
licorice root
cardamom

Often relied upon for easing digestive tension, Fennel supports comfort by encouraging gentle movement and relaxation within the gut.

CHICORY ROOT
cichorium intybus

flow

HOW SHE MIGHT HELP
Sluggish digestion, a sense of heaviness, and irregular appetite often benefit from Chicory, especially when digestive flow and liver support feel underactive.

WORKING WITH HER
Steady, moderate use allows Chicory's gently bitter and nourishing qualities to support digestion with balance. She is most often taken as a decoction or roasted root preparation and fits well into daily routines that encourage digestive rhythm. Ongoing relationship supports ease and regularity over time.

AVOID COMBINING
Chicory tends to work well on her own or alongside mild digestive herbs. Attentive use supports comfort when combining with strong bitters used in high amounts, as her bitter nature already engages digestive stimulation.

IMPORTANT NOTES
Chicory suits gradual, consistent use and is generally well tolerated. Careful attention supports those sensitive to bitter flavors, and beginning gently allows the body's response to guide continued relationship.

COMMON PREPARATIONS*

Tea (decoction)
Roasted root beverage
Tincture

*See the Preparation Guide in the back of this book

WORKS WELL WITH

dandelion root
gentian root
ginger root
peppermint
fennel seeds

Often valued for supporting digestive flow and liver function, Chicory helps the body engage nourishment with greater steadiness and balance.

TRIPHALA
emblica officinalis
terminalia chebula
terminalia bellirica

HOW SHE MIGHT HELP
Irregular digestion, sluggish elimination, and imbalance across the gut often benefit from Triphala, especially when support is needed for both movement and nourishment together.

WORKING WITH HER
Steady, consistent use allows Triphala's balancing nature to express itself clearly. She is most often taken as a powder, tablet, or infusion and fits well into daily routines focused on digestive regulation. Ongoing relationship supports regularity without harsh stimulation.

AVOID COMBINING
Triphala tends to serve best when not layered with strong laxatives or aggressively stimulating digestive remedies. Attentive use supports comfort when combining with other formulas that strongly influence elimination.

IMPORTANT NOTES
Triphala offers a gently cleansing yet nourishing profile and suits ongoing use. Beginning with modest amounts supports clear observation of the body's response, particularly for those sensitive to increased elimination.

---

regulate

COMMON PREPARATIONS*

Powder
Tablet or capsule
Tea (infusion)

*See the Preparation Guide in the back of this book

WORKS WELL WITH

ginger root
licorice root
fennel seeds
turmeric root
dandelion root

Known for harmonizing digestion through gentle regulation, Triphala supports balance across the gut while encouraging steady, comfortable elimination.

DANDELION ROOT
cichorium intybus

support

HOW SHE MIGHT HELP
Digestive sluggishness, a sense of fullness, and imbalance tied to liver congestion often ease with Dandelion, especially when elimination and appetite need gentle support.

WORKING WITH HER
Regular, steady use allows Dandelion's supportive and clearing qualities to unfold. She is most often taken as a decoction, tincture, or roasted root beverage and fits well into daily routines that encourage digestive flow and liver function. Consistent relationship supports balance and regularity over time.

AVOID COMBINING
Dandelion generally blends well with many digestive and liver-supporting herbs. Attentive use supports comfort when combining with strong diuretics or highly stimulating bitters used in large amounts.

IMPORTANT NOTES
Dandelion suits ongoing use and is widely well tolerated. Thoughtful attention serves those with bile duct or gallbladder considerations, and beginning gently allows the body's response to guide continued relationship.

COMMON PREPARATIONS*

Tea (decoction)
Roasted root beverage
Tincture

*See the Preparation Guide in the back of this book

WORKS WELL WITH
chicory root
ginger root
peppermint
fennel seeds
turmeric root

Long relied upon for supporting digestion and liver balance, Dandelion helps the body process nourishment with clarity and steady ease.

TURMERIC
curcuma longa

balance

HOW SHE MIGHT HELP
Digestive discomfort linked to strain, inflammation, or stagnation often responds well to Turmeric, especially when the gut and liver benefit from steady, warming support.

WORKING WITH HER
Consistent, mindful use allows Turmeric's supportive qualities to unfold gradually. She is most often taken as a powder, tincture, or infusion and integrates well into daily routines that emphasize digestive resilience. Ongoing relationship supports comfort and balance over time.

AVOID COMBINING
Turmeric serves best when used thoughtfully alongside other warming or strongly stimulating herbs. Careful attention also supports those working with anticoagulant medications, as her effects may feel more pronounced together.

IMPORTANT NOTES
Turmeric carries a warming, drying nature and suits measured use. Beginning gently supports clear observation of the body's response, particularly for those sensitive to heat or dryness within digestion.

COMMON PREPARATIONS*

Powder
Tincture
Tea (infusion or decoction)
Honey-based preparations

*See the Preparation Guide in the back of this book

WORKS WELL WITH

ginger root
dandelion root
licorice root
fennel seeds
black pepper

Valued for supporting digestive comfort and internal balance, Turmeric helps the body engage nourishment while easing inflammatory strain.

LICORICE ROOT
glycyrrhiza glabra

soothe

HOW SHE MIGHT HELP
Digestive irritation, dryness, and discomfort linked to inflammation often ease with Licorice, especially when the gut benefits from soothing and moisture-restoring support.

WORKING WITH HER
Gentle, measured use allows Licorice's harmonizing qualities to support digestion with steadiness. She is most often taken as a decoction, tincture, or powder and fits well into routines focused on calming and protecting digestive tissues. Ongoing relationship supports comfort and balance.

AVOID COMBINING
Licorice tends to work best when not layered heavily with other herbs that strongly influence fluid balance or blood pressure. Thoughtful attention also serves when combining with formulas designed for long-term use.

IMPORTANT NOTES
Licorice carries a moistening, tonifying nature and suits moderate use. Careful attention supports those with blood pressure considerations, and beginning gently allows the body's response to guide continued relationship.

COMMON PREPARATIONS*

Tea (decoction)
Tincture
Powder
Honey-based preparations

*See the Preparation Guide in the back of this book

WORKS WELL WITH

marshmallow root
slippery elm
ginger root
fennel seeds
turmeric root

Often chosen for its ability to soothe and unify digestive function, Licorice supports the gut by restoring comfort and internal harmony.

ACTIVATED CHARCOAL
glycyrrhiza glabra

relief

HOW SHE MIGHT HELP

Digestive distress marked by gas, bloating, or exposure to unwanted substances sometimes calls for Activated Charcoal, especially when binding and removal support feels appropriate.

WORKING WITH HER

Occasional, intentional use allows Activated Charcoal's absorptive qualities to serve digestion effectively. She is most often taken as a capsule or powder mixed with water and is traditionally used short term rather than as part of daily routine. Thoughtful timing supports clarity of effect.

AVOID COMBINING

Activated Charcoal serves best when taken apart from foods, supplements, and medications, as her binding nature may reduce their absorption. Attentive spacing also supports balance when working alongside other remedies intended for nourishment or tonification.

IMPORTANT NOTES

Activated Charcoal is suited for short-term use rather than ongoing support. Adequate hydration supports comfort, and careful attention is encouraged for those managing chronic digestive conditions or regular medication use.

COMMON PREPARATIONS*

Capsule
Powder mixed with water

*See the Preparation Guide in the back of this book

WORKS WELL WITH

ginger root
peppermint
fennel seeds
chamomile
plantain leaf

Used with intention and restraint, Activated Charcoal supports digestive relief by binding and carrying away what no longer serves the system.

BITTERS
blend of bitter herbs

awaken

HOW SHE MIGHT HELP
Low appetite, sluggish digestion, and a sense of heaviness before or after meals often respond to Bitters, especially when digestive readiness and flow need encouragement.

WORKING WITH HER
Intentional, measured use allows Bitters to stimulate digestive signaling with clarity. She is most often taken as a liquid formula shortly before meals and works best when approached as a supportive ritual rather than a constant companion. Regular use supports digestive engagement and awareness over time.

AVOID COMBINING
Bitters serve best when not layered with other strong bitter remedies used in high amounts. Careful attention also supports those experiencing active gastric irritation, as stimulation may feel intense when tissues are already inflamed.

IMPORTANT NOTES
Bitters emphasize stimulation rather than soothing and suit mindful use. Beginning gently supports awareness of the body's response, particularly for those sensitive to digestive activation or acidity.

COMMON PREPARATIONS*

Liquid bitters formula
Tincture blends

*See the Preparation Guide in the back of this book

WORKS WELL WITH
gentian root
chicory root
dandelion root
ginger root
fennel seeds

By awakening digestive awareness through taste and signaling, Bitters help the body prepare to receive nourishment with greater efficiency and balance.

MARSHMALLOW ROOT
althaea officinalis

soothe

HOW SHE MIGHT HELP
Dryness, irritation, and sensitivity along the digestive tract often ease with Marshmallow, especially when tissues benefit from gentle coating and moisture.

WORKING WITH HER
Slow, steady preparation allows Marshmallow's demulcent qualities to unfold fully. She is most often taken as a cold infusion or decoction and fits well into routines focused on soothing and protecting delicate digestive tissues. Consistent use supports comfort and resilience over time.

AVOID COMBINING
Marshmallow tends to serve best when taken apart from medications or supplements, as her coating nature may reduce absorption when used together. Thoughtful timing supports clarity and effectiveness.

IMPORTANT NOTES
Marshmallow is generally well tolerated and suits ongoing support for irritated tissues. Beginning gently allows the body's response to guide continued relationship, particularly when sensitivity is present.

COMMON PREPARATIONS*

Cold infusion
Tea (decoction)
Powder

*See the Preparation Guide in the back of this book

WORKS WELL WITH

slippery elm
plantain leaf
licorice root
chamomile
peppermint

Known for her deeply soothing presence, Marshmallow supports digestive comfort by protecting and restoring vulnerable tissues.

SLIPPERY ELM
ulmus rubra

calm

HOW SHE MIGHT HELP
Digestive irritation, dryness, and discomfort that arise from sensitive or compromised tissues often find relief with Slippery Elm, especially when soothing and protection are needed together.

WORKING WITH HER
Gentle, consistent use allows Slippery Elm's demulcent qualities to support digestive comfort. She is most often taken as a gruel, powder mixed with liquid, or infusion and fits well into routines focused on calming and restoring the gut lining. Ongoing relationship supports ease and resilience.

AVOID COMBINING
Slippery Elm is best taken apart from medications or supplements, as her coating nature may interfere with absorption when used at the same time. Thoughtful timing supports clarity and effectiveness.

IMPORTANT NOTES
Slippery Elm suits ongoing support for irritated tissues and is generally well tolerated. Beginning gently allows the body's response to guide continued relationship, particularly during periods of heightened sensitivity.

COMMON PREPARATIONS*

Powder mixed with water
Gruel or porridge
Infusion

*See the Preparation Guide in the back of this book

WORKS WELL WITH

marshmallow root
plantain leaf
licorice root
chamomile
peppermint

Valued for her protective and restorative qualities, Slippery Elm supports digestive comfort by cushioning and strengthening vulnerable tissues.

PEPPERMINT
mentha × piperita

settle

HOW SHE MIGHT HELP

Digestive tension, cramping, and discomfort linked to gas or spasms often ease with Peppermint, especially when the gut benefits from gentle relaxation and release.

WORKING WITH HER

Light, attentive use allows Peppermint's cooling and carminative qualities to support digestion with clarity. She is most often taken as an infusion, tincture, or aromatic preparation and fits well into routines that follow meals or moments of digestive strain. Regular relationship supports comfort and ease.

AVOID COMBINING

Peppermint serves best when not layered heavily with other strongly cooling or stimulating herbs used in high amounts. Thoughtful attention also supports those experiencing reflux, as her relaxing effect on tissues may feel less supportive in that context.

IMPORTANT NOTES

Peppermint is generally well tolerated and suits gentle, as-needed use. Beginning with modest amounts supports awareness of the body's response, particularly for those sensitive to cooling or aromatic herbs.

COMMON PREPARATIONS*

Tea (infusion)
Tincture
Essential oil (aromatic use)

*See the Preparation Guide in the back of this book

WORKS WELL WITH

fennel seeds
ginger root
chamomile
marshmallow root
licorice root

Often reached for when digestion feels tight or unsettled, Peppermint supports comfort by easing tension and restoring a sense of flow within the gut.

SECTION THREE
RESPIRATORY & IMMUNE SUPPORT

Immune health reflects the body's ongoing relationship with its environment, responding constantly to seasonal shifts, exposure, stress, and recovery. The respiratory system serves as both gateway and guardian, filtering what enters while supporting circulation, oxygenation, and defense. When these systems feel supported, the body often meets challenge with greater steadiness and resilience.

The plants gathered here offer a wide spectrum of immune and respiratory support. Some strengthen foundational defenses and build long-term resilience, while others focus on acute response, helping the body mobilize when strain or exposure arises. Several soothe irritated tissues, support clear breathing, or encourage the release of congestion, illustrating how protection and repair work together. Others nourish and tone, supporting recovery after periods of depletion or repeated demand.

Leaves, berries, roots, fungi, and flowers appear throughout these pages because of their familiarity and practical use across cultures and traditions. Together, they demonstrate core immune patterns such as warming and cooling, moistening and drying, stimulating and fortifying. Working with them reveals how immune strength is shaped through consistency, timing, and attentiveness rather than force.

These pages invite seasonal awareness and thoughtful observation. Attention to breath, circulation, and response becomes a way of listening, guided by plants that have long supported the body's capacity to adapt and defend. May this collection offer a steady entry point into immune and respiratory care and deepen understanding of the relationships that support vitality through changing conditions.

- elderberry
- astragalus
- marshmallow
- elderflower
- echinacea
- sage leaf
- rosemary
- peppermint
- spearmint
- mullein
- calendula
- hibiscus
- schisandra
- ginger
- chaga
- thyme
- oregano
- licorice root
- rosehips
- garlic
- tusli

ELDERBERRY
sambucus nigra

protect

HOW SHE MIGHT HELP

Periods of lowered immunity, seasonal challenge, and recovery after illness often draw attention to Elderberry, especially when the body benefits from nourishment and protection together.

WORKING WITH HER

Consistent, supportive use allows Elderberry's strengthening qualities to unfold with steadiness. She is most often taken as a syrup, tincture, or decoction and fits well into routines focused on immune support during times of increased exposure. Ongoing relationship supports resilience and recovery.

AVOID COMBINING

Elderberry tends to serve best when worked with on her own or alongside gentle immune-supportive herbs. Thoughtful attention supports balance when combining with strong stimulating remedies used in high amounts.

IMPORTANT NOTES

Elderberry is traditionally used in cooked or prepared form rather than raw. Regular, moderate use supports immune tone, and beginning gently allows the body's response to guide continued relationship.

COMMON PREPARATIONS*

Syrup
Tincture
Tea (decoction)

*See the Preparation Guide in the back of this book

WORKS WELL WITH

elderflower
rosehips
ginger
echinacea
tulsi (holy basil)

Known for supporting immune resilience through nourishment and protection, Elderberry helps the body meet seasonal demands with greater strength and ease.

ASTRAGALUS
astragalus membranaceus

strengthen

HOW SHE MIGHT HELP

Long-term immune depletion, frequent susceptibility, and fatigue tied to ongoing stress often benefit from Astragalus, especially when the body needs steady strengthening rather than acute intervention.

WORKING WITH HER

Consistent, long-view use allows Astragalus's fortifying qualities to build gradually. She is most often taken as a decoction, powder, or tincture and fits well into daily routines focused on immune tone and vitality. Ongoing relationship supports endurance and recovery over time.

AVOID COMBINING

Astragalus is best approached apart from acute immune stimulants used during active infection, as her role centers on building rather than mobilizing. Thoughtful attention also serves when layering with other strong tonics used in high amounts.

IMPORTANT NOTES

Astragalus suits steady, ongoing use and is generally well tolerated. Beginning gently supports clear observation of the body's response, particularly for those sensitive to tonifying herbs.

COMMON PREPARATIONS*

Tea (decoction)
Powder
Tincture

*See the Preparation Guide in the back of this book

WORKS WELL WITH

schisandra berries
reishi mushroom
ginger
tulsi (holy basil)
licorice root

Often chosen for building lasting immune strength, Astragalus supports the body's capacity to adapt, restore, and remain resilient over time.

MARSHMALLOW ROOT

althaea officinalis

calm

HOW SHE MIGHT HELP

Dryness, irritation, and sensitivity within the respiratory tract often respond well to Marshmallow, especially when coughing, throat discomfort, or inflamed tissues need soothing and protection.

WORKING WITH HER

Slow, patient preparation allows Marshmallow's demulcent qualities to express themselves fully. She is most often taken as a cold infusion or gentle decoction and fits well into routines that focus on calming and restoring delicate respiratory tissues. Consistent use supports comfort and ease.

AVOID COMBINING

Marshmallow is best taken apart from medications or supplements, as her coating nature may interfere with absorption when used together. Thoughtful timing supports clarity and effectiveness.

IMPORTANT NOTES

Marshmallow suits ongoing support for irritated or sensitive tissues and is generally well tolerated. Beginning gently allows the body's response to guide continued relationship, particularly during periods of dryness or strain.

COMMON PREPARATIONS*

Cold infusion
Tea (decoction)
Powder

*See the Preparation Guide in the back of this book

WORKS WELL WITH

mullein
elderflower
licorice root
thyme
peppermint

Valued for her ability to calm and protect vulnerable tissues, Marshmallow supports respiratory comfort by restoring moisture and resilience.

ELDERFLOWER
sambucus nigra

ease

HOW SHE MIGHT HELP

Congestion, mild feverishness, and respiratory discomfort linked to seasonal challenge often soften with Elderflower, especially when the body benefits from gentle opening and release.

WORKING WITH HER

Light, consistent use allows Elderflower's opening and supportive qualities to come forward. She is most often taken as a warm infusion or tincture and fits well into routines that support circulation, perspiration, and respiratory ease. Ongoing relationship supports comfort and balance.

AVOID COMBINING

Elderflower tends to work best without heavy layering alongside other strongly stimulating remedies used in high amounts. Thoughtful attention supports balance when combining with formulas intended for intense heat or forceful action.

IMPORTANT NOTES

Elderflower suits short-term or seasonal use and is generally well tolerated. Beginning gently supports clear observation of the body's response, particularly during periods of acute congestion or sensitivity.

COMMON PREPARATIONS*

Tea (infusion)
Tincture
Steam inhalation

*See the Preparation Guide in the back of this book

WORKS WELL WITH

elderberry
peppermint
yarrow
ginger
rosehips

Often reached for during times of seasonal transition, Elderflower supports the body by easing congestion and encouraging gentle, restorative flow.

ECHINACEA
echinacea purpurea

protect

HOW SHE MIGHT HELP

Early signs of immune challenge, throat discomfort, and heightened vulnerability often respond to Echinacea, especially when the body benefits from prompt, activating support.

WORKING WITH HER

Timely, attentive use allows Echinacea's stimulating qualities to engage the immune response clearly. She is most often taken as a tincture or tea and is commonly reached for at the onset of symptoms rather than for long-term daily use. Short, focused periods of use support effectiveness.

AVOID COMBINING

Echinacea serves best when not layered with other strong immune stimulants used in high amounts at the same time. Thoughtful attention also supports balance when combining with long-term tonics, as her role centers on activation rather than building.

IMPORTANT NOTES

Echinacea is well suited for acute or short-term support rather than extended use. Beginning gently supports clear observation of the body's response, particularly for those sensitive to immune stimulation.

COMMON PREPARATIONS*

Tincture
Tea (infusion)
Glycerite

*See the Preparation Guide in the back of this book

WORKS WELL WITH

elderberry
ginger
thyme
sage leaf
rosehips

Often chosen at the first sign of immune strain, Echinacea supports the body's ability to respond swiftly and decisively.

SAGE LEAF
salvia officinalis

clarify

HOW SHE MIGHT HELP

Sore throat, excess moisture, and respiratory discomfort often benefit from Sage, especially when tissues feel boggy and clarity is needed in the upper respiratory tract.

WORKING WITH HER

Measured, intentional use allows Sage's drying and clarifying qualities to support balance. She is most often taken as an infusion, tincture, or gargle and fits well into short-term routines focused on throat comfort and respiratory hygiene. Thoughtful use supports steadiness without excess.

AVOID COMBINING

Sage tends to serve best when not layered heavily with other strongly drying or stimulating herbs used in high amounts. Attentive use also supports balance when combining with concentrated essential oil preparations.

IMPORTANT NOTES

Sage carries a warming, astringent nature and suits moderate, time-bound use. Beginning gently supports awareness of the body's response, particularly for those sensitive to dryness or stimulation.

COMMON PREPARATIONS*

Tea (infusion)
Tincture
Gargle

*See the Preparation Guide in the back of this book

WORKS WELL WITH

thyme
echinacea
elderflower
peppermint
honey

Often reached for when clarity and containment are needed, Sage supports respiratory comfort by firming tissues and restoring balance.

ROSEMARY
salvia rosmarinus

circulate

HOW SHE MIGHT HELP

Stagnant breath, heavy congestion, and a sense of dullness during immune challenge often respond to Rosemary, especially when warmth and circulation support clearer respiratory function.

WORKING WITH HER

Mindful, moderate use allows Rosemary's clarifying qualities to support both respiration and immune engagement. She is most often taken as an infusion, tincture, or steam preparation and fits well into short-term routines focused on opening and movement. Thoughtful relationship supports alert presence and clear breath.

AVOID COMBINING

Rosemary tends to feel most supportive when used apart from other strongly stimulating herbs taken in high amounts. Careful attention also serves when combining with substances that significantly increase heat or activation.

IMPORTANT NOTES

Rosemary carries a warming, aromatic nature and suits measured use. Beginning gently supports awareness of the body's response, particularly during periods of intensity or heightened stimulation.

COMMON PREPARATIONS*

Tea (infusion)
Tincture
Steam inhalation
Aromatic preparation

*See the Preparation Guide in the back of this book

WORKS WELL WITH

thyme
sage leaf
peppermint
elderflower
ginger

Through warmth and movement, Rosemary supports respiratory clarity and helps the body engage immune response with steadiness and focus.

PEPPERMINT
mentha x piperita

cool

HOW SHE MIGHT HELP

Tightness in the chest, irritated airways, and respiratory discomfort linked to congestion often ease with Peppermint, especially when cooling clarity and gentle opening are needed.

WORKING WITH HER

Light, attentive use allows Peppermint's cooling and dispersing qualities to support clear breathing. She is most often taken as an infusion, tincture, or aromatic preparation and fits well into short-term routines focused on easing congestion and restoring comfort. Thoughtful use supports relief without heaviness.

AVOID COMBINING

Peppermint tends to feel most balanced when not layered heavily with other strongly cooling or stimulating herbs used in high amounts. Careful attention also serves those experiencing reflux, as her relaxing effect on tissues may feel less supportive in that context.

IMPORTANT NOTES

Peppermint carries a cooling, aromatic nature and suits measured use. Beginning gently supports awareness of the body's response, particularly for those sensitive to cooling or mentholated herbs.

COMMON PREPARATIONS*

Tea (infusion)
Tincture
Steam inhalation
Aromatic preparation

*See the Preparation Guide in the back of this book

WORKS WELL WITH

elderflower
thyme
ginger
mullein
licorice root

By cooling and opening the airways, Peppermint supports easier breath and renewed respiratory comfort.

SPEARMINT
mentha spicata

refresh

HOW SHE MIGHT HELP

Mild congestion, throat irritation, and respiratory tension that benefit from gentle support often respond well to Spearmint, especially when a softer touch is preferred.

WORKING WITH HER

Gentle, consistent use allows Spearmint's refreshing qualities to support the respiratory system without intensity. She is most often taken as an infusion or tincture and fits comfortably into daily routines that favor ease and lightness. Ongoing relationship supports relaxed, steady breathing.

AVOID COMBINING

Spearmint generally integrates smoothly with other mild respiratory herbs. Attentive use supports balance when combining with stronger aromatic or cooling remedies used in high amounts.

IMPORTANT NOTES

Spearmint is typically well tolerated and suits gentle, ongoing use. Beginning moderately allows the body's response to guide continued relationship, particularly for those sensitive to stronger mints.

COMMON PREPARATIONS*

Tea (infusion)
Tincture
Fresh leaf preparations

*See the Preparation Guide in the back of this book

WORKS WELL WITH

elderflower
hibiscus
rosehips
lemon balm
mullein

With a softer aromatic presence, Spearmint supports respiratory ease by refreshing the breath and calming irritation.

MULLEIN
verbascum thapsus

HOW SHE MIGHT HELP

Dry cough, irritated airways, and lingering congestion often respond well to Mullein, especially when the lungs need soothing support and gentle clearing.

WORKING WITH HER

Patient, consistent use allows Mullein's softening qualities to support respiratory comfort. She is most often taken as an infusion or tincture and fits well into routines focused on calming irritation and encouraging productive breath. Ongoing relationship supports ease and openness within the lungs.

AVOID COMBINING

Mullein generally blends well with many respiratory herbs and tends to feel balanced on her own. Attentive preparation supports comfort, particularly when combining with very drying remedies used in high amounts.

IMPORTANT NOTES

Mullein suits gentle, ongoing use and is typically well tolerated. Careful straining of infusions supports throat comfort, and beginning gently allows the body's response to guide continued relationship.

---

soothe 40

COMMON PREPARATIONS*

Tea (infusion, well strained)
Tincture
Steam inhalation

*See the Preparation Guide in the back of this book

WORKS WELL WITH

marshmallow root
licorice root
elderflower
thyme
peppermint

Often turned to for quiet lung support, Mullein helps restore comfort by soothing irritation and encouraging freer breath.

CALENDULA
calendula officinalis

restore

HOW SHE MIGHT HELP

Inflamed tissues, sluggish lymphatic movement, and immune strain often benefit from Calendula flower, especially when gentle cleansing and repair are needed together.

WORKING WITH HER

Steady, attentive use allows Calendula's restorative qualities to support immune and respiratory health. She is most often taken as an infusion or tincture and fits well into routines that emphasize tissue healing and lymphatic flow. Consistent relationship supports recovery and balance.

AVOID COMBINING

Calendula generally integrates smoothly with a wide range of immune-supportive herbs. Thoughtful attention supports balance when combining with strongly stimulating remedies used in high amounts.

IMPORTANT NOTES

Calendula is well suited for ongoing use and is typically well tolerated. Beginning gently supports awareness of the body's response, particularly when working with sensitive or inflamed tissues.

COMMON PREPARATIONS*

Tea (infusion)
Tincture
Infused oil (external use)

*See the Preparation Guide in the back of this book

WORKS WELL WITH

elderflower
mullein
rosehips
licorice root
hibiscus

With a steady, restorative presence, Calendula supports immune balance by encouraging gentle cleansing and tissue repair.

HIBISCUS
hibiscus sabdariffa

cool

HOW SHE MIGHT HELP

Heat, inflammation, and immune strain often soften with Hibiscus, especially when the body benefits from cooling, hydration, and circulatory support.

WORKING WITH HER

Gentle, consistent use allows Hibiscus's cooling and tonifying qualities to support immune balance. She is most often taken as an infusion or blended beverage and fits well into routines that emphasize hydration and circulation. Ongoing relationship supports refreshment and resilience.

AVOID COMBINING

Hibiscus tends to feel most balanced when not layered heavily with other strongly cooling herbs used in high amounts. Thoughtful attention also serves when combining with remedies that significantly lower blood pressure.

IMPORTANT NOTES

Hibiscus carries a cooling, mildly astringent nature and suits measured use. Beginning gently supports awareness of the body's response, particularly for those sensitive to cooling or dryness.

COMMON PREPARATIONS*

Tea (infusion)
Cold infusion
Syrup or blended beverage

*See the Preparation Guide in the back of this book

WORKS WELL WITH

rosehips
elderflower
spearmint
ginger
hibiscus blends well with warming companions

With a bright, cooling presence, Hibiscus supports immune balance by refreshing circulation and easing inflammatory strain.

SCHISANDRA BERRIES
schisandra chinensis

strengthen

HOW SHE MIGHT HELP

Immune fatigue, respiratory weakness, and reduced resilience during prolonged stress often benefit from Schisandra, especially when endurance and adaptability feel diminished.

WORKING WITH HER

Steady, intentional use allows Schisandra's tonifying qualities to build over time. She is most often taken as a decoction, tincture, or powder and fits well into routines that support lung strength and immune resilience. Ongoing relationship supports balance under sustained demand.

AVOID COMBINING

Schisandra tends to serve best when used apart from other strong tonics taken in high amounts at the same time. Thoughtful attention also supports those working with medications that strongly influence liver metabolism.

IMPORTANT NOTES

Schisandra carries a concentrated, astringent nature and suits measured, consistent use. Beginning gently supports clear observation of the body's response, particularly for those sensitive to stimulation or tightening effects.

COMMON PREPARATIONS*

Tea (decoction)
Tincture
Powder

*See the Preparation Guide in the back of this book

WORKS WELL WITH

astragalus
reishi mushroom
licorice root
ginger
tulsi (holy basil)

By strengthening resilience at a deep level, Schisandra supports the lungs and immune system in meeting sustained challenge with steadiness and clarity.

GINGER
zingiber officinale

warm

HOW SHE MIGHT HELP
Chill, congestion, and sluggish immune response often shift with Ginger, especially when warmth and circulation support respiratory comfort.

WORKING WITH HER
Moderate, intentional use allows Ginger's warming qualities to support both immunity and breath. She is most often taken as a fresh infusion, decoction, tincture, or powder and fits well into short-term routines during seasonal challenge. Consistent use supports movement and clarity.

AVOID COMBINING
Ginger tends to feel most balanced when not layered heavily with other strongly heating herbs used in high amounts. Thoughtful attention also supports comfort for those sensitive to warmth or intensity.

IMPORTANT NOTES
Ginger carries an activating, warming nature and suits measured use. Beginning gently supports awareness of the body's response, particularly during periods of heat or inflammation.

COMMON PREPARATIONS*

Tea (infusion or decoction)
Fresh juice
Tincture
Powder

*See the Preparation Guide in the back of this book

WORKS WELL WITH

elderberry
thyme
licorice root
peppermint
garlic

Through warmth and circulation, Ginger supports immune response and encourages freer movement within the respiratory system.

CHAGA
inonotus obliquus

nourish

HOW SHE MIGHT HELP

Immune depletion, inflammation, and prolonged strain often respond to Chaga, especially when the body benefits from deep nourishment and steady resilience.

WORKING WITH HER

Long-view, consistent use allows Chaga's grounding qualities to build gradually. She is most often taken as a decoction, powder, or tincture and fits well into routines focused on immune endurance and recovery. Ongoing relationship supports balance over time.

AVOID COMBINING

Chaga tends to serve best when used thoughtfully alongside other tonics. Attentive use supports balance for those working with immune-modulating remedies used in high amounts.

IMPORTANT NOTES

Chaga carries a dense, strengthening nature and suits steady use rather than acute response. Beginning gently supports clear observation of the body's response, particularly for those sensitive to concentrated tonics.

COMMON PREPARATIONS*

Tea (decoction)
Powder
Tincture

*See the Preparation Guide in the back of this book

WORKS WELL WITH

astragalus
schisandra berries
rosehips
licorice root
ginger

By nourishing immune strength at a foundational level, Chaga supports resilience through periods of ongoing demand.

THYME
thymus vulgaris

open

HOW SHE MIGHT HELP

Chest congestion, cough, and respiratory discomfort often ease with Thyme, especially when clearing and antimicrobial support are needed together.

WORKING WITH HER

Focused, time-bound use allows Thyme's aromatic and protective qualities to support the lungs. She is most often taken as an infusion, tincture, or steam preparation and fits well into short-term routines during acute respiratory challenge. Thoughtful use supports clarity and relief.

AVOID COMBINING

Thyme tends to feel most supportive when not layered heavily with other strongly stimulating or drying herbs used in high amounts. Careful attention also serves when combining with concentrated essential oil preparations.

IMPORTANT NOTES

Thyme carries a warming, aromatic nature and suits measured use. Beginning gently supports awareness of the body's response, particularly for those sensitive to intensity or dryness.

COMMON PREPARATIONS*

Tea (infusion)
Tincture
Steam inhalation

*See the Preparation Guide in the back of this book

WORKS WELL WITH

sage leaf
mullein
ginger
elderberry
licorice root

With a clarifying and protective presence, Thyme supports respiratory comfort by helping the body release congestion and restore ease of breath.

OREGANO
origanum vulgare

clarify

HOW SHE MIGHT HELP

Acute respiratory challenge, congestion, and immune strain often call for Oregano, especially when strong antimicrobial support and warmth are needed together.

WORKING WITH HER

Focused, time-bound use allows Oregano's potent qualities to engage the immune system clearly. She is most often taken as an infusion, tincture, or diluted aromatic preparation and fits well into short-term routines during periods of active challenge. Attentive use supports effectiveness without excess.

AVOID COMBINING

Oregano tends to feel most balanced when not layered heavily with other strongly heating or stimulating herbs used in high amounts. Thoughtful attention also supports comfort when combining with concentrated essential oil preparations.

IMPORTANT NOTES

Oregano carries a strong, warming nature and suits short-term use. Beginning gently supports awareness of the body's response, particularly for those sensitive to heat or intensity.

COMMON PREPARATIONS*

Tea (infusion)
Tincture
Steam inhalation

*See the Preparation Guide in the back of this book

WORKS WELL WITH

thyme
garlic
elderberry
ginger
licorice root

With a bold and protective character, Oregano supports immune response by helping the body address active challenge with strength and clarity.

LICORICE ROOT
glycyrrhiza glabra

comfort

HOW SHE MIGHT HELP

Irritated airways, dry cough, and immune fatigue often benefit from Licorice, especially when soothing, moistening, and harmonizing support is needed.

WORKING WITH HER

Gentle, measured use allows Licorice's balancing qualities to support respiratory comfort. She is most often taken as a decoction, tincture, or powder and fits well into routines that emphasize tissue protection and recovery. Ongoing relationship supports steadiness and ease.

AVOID COMBINING

Licorice tends to serve best when not layered heavily with other herbs that strongly influence fluid balance or blood pressure. Thoughtful attention also serves when combining with long-term formulas.

IMPORTANT NOTES

Licorice carries a moistening, tonifying nature and suits moderate use. Careful attention supports those with blood pressure considerations, and beginning gently allows the body's response to guide continued relationship.

COMMON PREPARATIONS*

Tea (decoction)
Tincture
Powder

*See the Preparation Guide in the back of this book

WORKS WELL WITH

mullein
marshmallow root
thyme
elderflower
rosehips

By calming irritation and unifying immune response, Licorice supports the respiratory system in restoring comfort and balance.

ROSEHIPS
rosa canina

strengthen

HOW SHE MIGHT HELP

Immune fatigue, seasonal vulnerability, and recovery after illness often respond to Rosehips, especially when nourishment and gentle strengthening are needed.

WORKING WITH HER

Consistent, supportive use allows Rosehips' nutritive qualities to build steadily. She is most often taken as an infusion, powder, or syrup and fits well into daily routines focused on immune resilience. Ongoing relationship supports vitality and recovery.

AVOID COMBINING

Rosehips tend to work most smoothly when taken separately from high-dose iron supplements, as their vitamin C content can increase iron absorption. Attentive pacing also supports balance when layering with very acidic preparations used in large amounts, particularly for sensitive digestion.

IMPORTANT NOTES

Rosehips offer a cooling, mildly astringent profile and suit ongoing use. Careful straining of infusions supports throat comfort, and beginning gently allows the body's response to guide continued relationship.

COMMON PREPARATIONS*

Tea (infusion, well strained)
Powder
Syrup

*See the Preparation Guide in the back of this book

WORKS WELL WITH

elderberry
hibiscus
elderflower
licorice root
tulsi (holy basil)

Through gentle nourishment and steady strengthening, Rosehips support immune resilience and recovery across changing seasons.

GARLIC
allium sativum

protect

HOW SHE MIGHT HELP

Acute immune challenge, congestion, and respiratory strain often call for Garlic, especially when strong protective support and circulation are needed together.

WORKING WITH HER

Intentional, time-limited use allows Garlic's potent qualities to engage immune response effectively. She is most often taken fresh, as a tincture, or infused into food and fits well into short-term routines during periods of active challenge. Thoughtful use supports strength without overwhelm.

AVOID COMBINING

Garlic tends to feel most balanced when not layered heavily with other strongly heating or stimulating herbs used in high amounts. Attentive use also supports those working with anticoagulant medications, as her effects may feel more pronounced together.

IMPORTANT NOTES

Garlic carries a strong, warming nature and suits focused use rather than ongoing daily reliance. Beginning gently supports awareness of the body's response, particularly for those sensitive to heat or intensity.

COMMON PREPARATIONS*

Fresh clove
Tincture
Honey infusion
Food-based preparations

*See the Preparation Guide in the back of this book

WORKS WELL WITH

thyme
oregano
ginger
elderberry
licorice root

Through warmth and decisive action, Garlic supports immune defense and helps the body respond clearly during times of challenge.

TULSI
(HOLY BASIL)

ocimum sanctum

balance

HOW SHE MIGHT HELP

Immune stress, respiratory vulnerability, and fatigue shaped by ongoing pressure often benefit from Tulsi, especially when resilience and balance are needed together.

WORKING WITH HER

Gentle, consistent use allows Tulsi's harmonizing qualities to support both immunity and the nervous system. She is most often taken as an infusion, tincture, or powder and fits comfortably into daily routines focused on steady support. Ongoing relationship supports adaptability and recovery.

AVOID COMBINING

Tulsi generally integrates smoothly with a wide range of immune-supportive herbs. Thoughtful attention supports balance when combining with strong stimulating remedies used in high amounts.

IMPORTANT NOTES

Tulsi suits ongoing use and is typically well tolerated. Beginning gently supports clear observation of the body's response, particularly during periods of sustained stress or depletion.

COMMON PREPARATIONS*

Tea (infusion)
Tincture
Powder

*See the Preparation Guide in the back of this book

WORKS WELL WITH

elderberry
astragalus
ginger
rosehips
licorice root

By supporting resilience across body and breath, Tulsi helps the immune system respond with steadiness and grace.

SECTION FOUR
INFLAMMATION & PAIN SUPPORT

Pain and inflammation reflect how the body responds to strain, injury, repetition, and repair. These signals arise through movement, stillness, impact, and overuse, offering information about tissues, circulation, and recovery. When inflammation is supported thoughtfully, the body often regains comfort, mobility, and trust in its own capacity to heal.

The remedies gathered here approach pain and inflammation from multiple directions. Some encourage circulation and warmth, helping ease stiffness and restore movement. Others calm irritated tissues, soften guarding, or support the release of tension held within muscles, joints, and connective structures. Several work more deeply, nourishing repair processes and supporting long-term resilience where chronic discomfort has taken hold. Together, they illustrate how relief and restoration unfold through both immediate support and steady care.

Roots, barks, leaves, minerals, and topical preparations appear throughout these pages because of their long-standing use and practical relevance. They demonstrate core patterns of pain support such as warming and cooling, dispersing and grounding, soothing and strengthening. Working with them reveals how inflammation responds to timing, consistency, and respectful engagement rather than forceful intervention.

These pages invite close attention to sensation, movement, and recovery. Noticing how pain shifts, settles, or signals change becomes a form of listening guided by plants and remedies that have long supported the body's ability to mend and adapt. May this collection offer a grounded entry point into pain and inflammation care and deepen understanding of the relationships that support comfort, mobility, and sustained ease.

- comfrey
- solomon's seal
- msm
- devil's claw
- wild yam root
- boswellia
- ginger
- magnesium
- cayenne
- burdock root
- turmeric
- skullcap
- cleavers
- chamomile
- lemon balm
- white willow

COMFREY (TOPICAL)

symphytum officinale

comfort

HOW SHE MIGHT HELP

Localized pain, bruising, strains, and tissue discomfort often respond well to Comfrey, especially when support for repair and soothing is needed at the surface level.

WORKING WITH HER

Topical, attentive application allows Comfrey's restorative qualities to support tissue comfort and recovery. She is most often used as a salve, poultice, or infused oil and fits well into routines that focus on supporting healing after strain or injury. Consistent external use supports ease and resilience.

AVOID COMBINING

Comfrey serves best when applied to clean, intact skin without layering alongside other strong topical stimulants. Thoughtful use supports clarity when combining with warming or circulatory remedies used externally.

IMPORTANT NOTES

Comfrey is traditionally reserved for external use due to her strong tissue-building nature. Application supports short-term recovery rather than prolonged or open-ended use, and careful attention serves when working near broken skin.

COMMON PREPARATIONS*

Salve
Infused oil
Poultice
Compress

*See the Preparation Guide in the back of this book

WORKS WELL WITH

calendula flower
plantain leaf
chamomile
arnica (topical)
lavender

Through steady, surface-level support, Comfrey encourages comfort and repair where tissues have been strained or unsettled.

SOLOMON'S SEAL ROOT
polygonatum biflorum

balance

HOW SHE MIGHT HELP

Joint discomfort, connective tissue strain, and pain linked to misalignment or overuse often benefit from Solomon's Seal, especially when stability and restoration are needed together.

WORKING WITH HER

Steady, patient use allows Solomon's Seal's supportive qualities to engage deep tissues over time. She is most often taken as a tincture or decoction and fits well into routines that emphasize gradual repair and improved range of motion. Ongoing relationship supports resilience within joints and connective structures.

AVOID COMBINING

Solomon's Seal tends to serve best when not layered heavily with strongly dispersing or aggressively stimulating remedies used in high amounts. Thoughtful attention supports balance when combining with formulas intended for long-term structural support.

IMPORTANT NOTES

Solomon's Seal carries a grounding, restorative nature and suits consistent, moderate use. Beginning gently supports clear observation of the body's response, particularly when working with chronic or long-standing patterns of discomfort.

COMMON PREPARATIONS*

Tincture
Tea (decoction)

*See the Preparation Guide in the back of this book

WORKS WELL WITH

devil's claw
turmeric
ginger
skullcap
burdock root

Through slow, deliberate support of connective tissues, Solomon's Seal helps restore balance, strength, and ease of movement over time.

MSM
methylsulfonylmethane

ease

HOW MSM MIGHT HELP

Joint stiffness, muscular soreness, and discomfort linked to inflammation often ease with MSM, especially when tissues benefit from added flexibility and support for repair.

WORKING WITH MSM

Gradual, consistent use allows MSM's supportive qualities to build steadily. She is most often taken as a powder or capsule and fits well into daily routines focused on joint comfort and mobility. Ongoing relationship supports resilience within connective tissues.

AVOID COMBINING

MSM generally integrates smoothly with many anti-inflammatory remedies. Attentive use supports balance when combining with other sulfur-containing supplements used in high amounts.

IMPORTANT NOTES

MSM suits ongoing use and is typically well tolerated. Beginning with a modest amount supports awareness of the body's response, particularly during the first weeks of use.

COMMON PREPARATIONS*

Powder
Capsule

*See the Preparation Guide in the back of this book

WORKS WELL WITH

turmeric
ginger
magnesium
boswellia
solomon's seal root

By supporting tissue flexibility and repair, MSM helps the body move with greater ease and comfort.

DEVIL'S CLAW
harpagophytum procumbens

mobility

56

HOW SHE MIGHT HELP

Persistent joint pain, inflammation, and discomfort tied to chronic strain often respond to Devil's Claw, especially when deeper relief and mobility support are needed.

WORKING WITH HER

Measured, consistent use allows Devil's Claw's anti-inflammatory qualities to express themselves clearly. She is most often taken as a tincture, capsule, or decoction and fits well into routines addressing ongoing musculoskeletal discomfort. Ongoing relationship supports improved movement over time.

AVOID COMBINING

Devil's Claw tends to serve best when not layered heavily with other strong anti-inflammatory or bitter remedies used in high amounts. Thoughtful attention also supports those with sensitive digestion.

IMPORTANT NOTES

Devil's Claw carries a strong, focused character and suits steady rather than short-term use. Beginning gently supports clear observation of the body's response, particularly for those new to bitter herbs.

COMMON PREPARATIONS*

Tincture
Capsule
Tea (decoction)

*See the Preparation Guide in the back of this book

WORKS WELL WITH

turmeric
ginger
solomon's seal root
boswellia
burdock root

Through deep anti-inflammatory support, Devil's Claw helps restore comfort and mobility where pain has become persistent.

WILD YAM ROOT
dioscorea villosa

calm

HOW SHE MIGHT HELP

Muscular cramping, spasms, and pain shaped by tension or hormonal fluctuation often soften with Wild Yam, especially when the body seeks relaxation and ease.

WORKING WITH HER

Gentle, attentive use allows Wild Yam's antispasmodic qualities to support comfort. She is most often taken as a tincture or decoction and fits well into routines focused on easing muscular tension and calming inflammation. Consistent relationship supports release and balance.

AVOID COMBINING

Wild Yam generally integrates smoothly with many pain-supportive herbs. Attentive use supports balance when combining with strong sedative remedies used in high amounts.

IMPORTANT NOTES

Wild Yam suits moderate, ongoing use and is typically well tolerated. Beginning gently supports awareness of the body's response, particularly for those sensitive to shifts in muscle tone or relaxation.

COMMON PREPARATIONS*

Tincture
Tea (decoction)

*See the Preparation Guide in the back of this book

WORKS WELL WITH

skullcap
ginger
turmeric
chamomile
lemon balm

By easing tension and calming spasm, Wild Yam supports the body in finding relief and softness where pain has taken hold.

BOSWELLIA
boswellia serrata

comfort

HOW SHE MIGHT HELP

Inflammation rooted in joints, connective tissues, and chronic strain often responds well to Boswellia, especially when swelling and stiffness limit comfortable movement.

WORKING WITH HER

Steady, consistent use allows Boswellia's resinous qualities to support inflammation balance over time. She is most often taken as a capsule, powder, or tincture and fits well into routines addressing ongoing discomfort and mobility concerns. Ongoing relationship supports gradual improvement in ease and range of motion.

AVOID COMBINING

Boswellia tends to serve best when not layered heavily with other concentrated anti-inflammatory supplements used in high amounts. Thoughtful attention supports comfort when combining with additional joint-focused formulas.

IMPORTANT NOTES

Boswellia carries a focused, tonifying nature and suits consistent use rather than acute intervention. Beginning gently supports clear observation of the body's response, particularly during longer-term use.

COMMON PREPARATIONS*

Capsule
Powder
Tincture

*See the Preparation Guide in the back of this book

WORKS WELL WITH

turmeric
ginger
devil's claw
msm
burdock root

By addressing inflammation at its source, Boswellia supports steadier movement and sustained joint comfort.

GINGER
zingiber officinale

warm

HOW SHE MIGHT HELP
Stiffness, soreness, and inflammation that benefit from warmth and circulation often ease with Ginger, especially when pain feels rooted in tension or stagnation.

WORKING WITH HER
Moderate, attentive use allows Ginger's warming qualities to support circulation and tissue comfort. She is most often taken as an infusion, decoction, tincture, or topical preparation and fits well into routines focused on loosening tight or guarded areas. Consistent relationship supports movement and relief.

AVOID COMBINING
Ginger tends to feel most balanced when not layered heavily with other strongly heating remedies used in high amounts. Thoughtful attention also supports comfort for those sensitive to warmth or intensity.

IMPORTANT NOTES
Ginger carries an activating nature and suits measured use. Beginning gently supports awareness of the body's response, particularly during periods of inflammation or heat.

COMMON PREPARATIONS*

Tea (infusion or decoction)
Tincture
Poultice or compress
Powder

*See the Preparation Guide in the back of this book

WORKS WELL WITH
turmeric
cayenne pepper
boswellia
devil's claw
magnesium

Through warmth and circulation, Ginger supports relief by helping tissues soften and release held tension.

IONIC MAGNESIUM
magnesium citrate

relax

HOW SHE MIGHT HELP

Muscle tension, cramping, and discomfort linked to nervous system strain or mineral depletion often respond to Magnesium, especially when relaxation and balance are needed together.

WORKING WITH HER

Gentle, consistent use allows Magnesium's calming qualities to support muscular and nervous system ease. She is most often taken in liquid ionic form and fits well into routines focused on relaxation, recovery, and sleep support. Ongoing relationship supports softness and release.

AVOID COMBINING

Magnesium generally integrates smoothly with many pain-supportive remedies. Attentive use supports comfort when combining with other mineral supplements used in high amounts.

IMPORTANT NOTES

Magnesium suits ongoing use and is typically well tolerated. Beginning with a modest amount supports awareness of the body's response, particularly in digestion and elimination.

COMMON PREPARATIONS*

Liquid ionic supplement

*See the Preparation Guide in the back of this book

WORKS WELL WITH

skullcap
chamomile
lemon balm
turmeric
ginger

By supporting relaxation at the muscular and nervous system level, Magnesium helps the body release tension and restore comfort.

CAYENNE PEPPER
capsicum annuum

warm

HOW SHE MIGHT HELP

Stiffness, circulatory stagnation, and pain that benefit from warmth and movement often respond to Cayenne, especially when tissues feel cold or bound.

WORKING WITH HER

Measured, intentional use allows Cayenne's stimulating qualities to support circulation and pain relief. She is most often taken in very small amounts internally or used topically in salves and liniments. Thoughtful use supports effectiveness without overwhelm.

AVOID COMBINING

Cayenne tends to serve best when not layered heavily with other strongly heating remedies used in high amounts. Attentive use also supports comfort for those sensitive to heat or irritation.

IMPORTANT NOTES

Cayenne carries a strong, activating nature and suits careful dosing. Beginning gently supports clear observation of the body's response, particularly when working internally.

COMMON PREPARATIONS*

Powder
Tincture
Salve or liniment

*See the Preparation Guide in the back of this book

WORKS WELL WITH

ginger
turmeric
boswellia
burdock root
magnesium

Through warmth and circulation, Cayenne supports pain relief by helping the body reestablish movement and flow.

BURDOCK ROOT
arctium lappa

clear

HOW SHE MIGHT HELP

Chronic inflammation, stiffness, and pain linked to systemic congestion often benefit from Burdock, especially when gentle cleansing and nourishment support recovery.

WORKING WITH HER

Steady, long-view use allows Burdock's supportive qualities to unfold gradually. She is most often taken as a decoction, tincture, or food-based preparation and fits well into routines focused on reducing inflammatory load. Ongoing relationship supports resilience and balance.

AVOID COMBINING

Burdock generally integrates smoothly with many pain- and inflammation-supportive herbs. Attentive use supports balance when combining with strong diuretics used in high amounts.

IMPORTANT NOTES

Burdock suits consistent, moderate use and is typically well tolerated. Beginning gently supports awareness of the body's response, particularly during periods of detoxification or transition.

COMMON PREPARATIONS*

Tea (decoction)
Tincture
Food-based preparations

*See the Preparation Guide in the back of this book

WORKS WELL WITH

turmeric
ginger
boswellia
devil's claw
cleavers

By supporting steady cleansing and nourishment, Burdock helps the body ease inflammation and restore comfort over time.

TURMERIC
curcuma longa

relieve

HOW SHE MIGHT HELP

Inflammation, joint discomfort, and pain shaped by systemic strain often respond well to Turmeric, especially when tissues benefit from steady, warming support.

WORKING WITH HER

Consistent, mindful use allows Turmeric's balancing qualities to unfold gradually. She is most often taken as a powder, tincture, or infusion and fits well into daily routines focused on long-term inflammation support. Ongoing relationship supports comfort and resilience over time.

AVOID COMBINING

Turmeric tends to serve best when used thoughtfully alongside other warming or strongly stimulating remedies. Attentive use also supports those working with anticoagulant medications, as effects may feel more pronounced together.

IMPORTANT NOTES

Turmeric carries a warming, drying nature and suits measured use. Beginning gently supports clear observation of the body's response, particularly for those sensitive to heat or dryness.

COMMON PREPARATIONS*

Powder
Tincture
Tea (infusion or decoction)
Honey-based preparations

*See the Preparation Guide in the back of this book

WORKS WELL WITH

ginger
boswellia
burdock root
magnesium
cayenne pepper

Through steady anti-inflammatory support, Turmeric helps the body soften pain and restore balance across joints and tissues.

SKULLCAP
scutellaria lateriflora

calm

HOW SHE MIGHT HELP
Pain intensified by nervous system tension, muscle guarding, or stress often eases with Skullcap, especially when relaxation and release support comfort.

WORKING WITH HER
Gentle, attentive use allows Skullcap's calming qualities to support both nerves and muscles. She is most often taken as a tincture or infusion and fits well into routines focused on easing tension and restoring ease. Ongoing relationship supports softness and steadiness.

AVOID COMBINING
Skullcap suits ongoing use and is generally well tolerated. Beginning gently supports awareness of the body's response, particularly when pain is closely tied to stress or nervous system activation.

IMPORTANT NOTES
Skullcap offers its greatest support through steady, consistent use rather than occasional dosing. Beginning with a low amount and observing response supports clarity, especially for those with heightened nervous system sensitivity. This plant carries a deeply calming influence and pairs well with rest, gentle movement, and periods of recovery.

COMMON PREPARATIONS*

Tincture
Tea (infusion)

*See the Preparation Guide in the back of this book

WORKS WELL WITH

magnesium
chamomile
lemon balm
wild yam root
turmeric

By calming the nervous system and easing muscular tension, Skullcap supports relief where pain is held through stress and strain.

CLEAVERS
galium aparine

release

HOW SHE MIGHT HELP

Inflammatory swelling, fluid retention, and discomfort linked to lymphatic congestion often benefit from Cleavers, especially when gentle movement and drainage support relief.

WORKING WITH HER

Steady, light use allows Cleavers' cooling and moving qualities to support lymphatic flow. She is most often taken as a fresh infusion or tincture and fits well into routines focused on reducing stagnation. Ongoing relationship supports softness and release.

AVOID COMBINING

Cleavers generally integrates smoothly with many inflammation-supportive herbs. Attentive use supports balance when combining with strong diuretics used in high amounts.

IMPORTANT NOTES

Cleavers carries a cooling, moistening nature and suits gentle, ongoing use. Beginning gently supports clear observation of the body's response, particularly for those sensitive to cooling effects.

COMMON PREPARATIONS*

Tea (infusion)
Tincture
Fresh juice

*See the Preparation Guide in the back of this book

WORKS WELL WITH

burdock root
calendula flower
turmeric
lemon balm
chamomile

By encouraging lymphatic movement and easing congestion, Cleavers supports the body in releasing inflammation and restoring comfort.

CHAMOMILE
matricaria chamomilla

calm

HOW SHE MIGHT HELP

Pain shaped by tension, inflammation, or digestive distress often softens with Chamomile, especially when the body benefits from calming and gentle anti-inflammatory support.

WORKING WITH HER

Consistent, soothing use allows Chamomile's calming qualities to support both muscles and tissues. She is most often taken as an infusion or tincture and fits well into routines focused on easing discomfort and restoring relaxation. Ongoing relationship supports comfort and softness.

AVOID COMBINING

Chamomile generally integrates smoothly with many pain-supportive herbs. Attentive use supports balance when combining with stronger sedative remedies used in high amounts.

IMPORTANT NOTES

Chamomile suits gentle, ongoing use and is typically well tolerated. Beginning gently supports awareness of the body's response, particularly for those sensitive to plants in the daisy family.

COMMON PREPARATIONS*

Tea (infusion)
Tincture
Compress

*See the Preparation Guide in the back of this book

WORKS WELL WITH

lemon balm
skullcap
wild yam root
ginger
cleavers

By calming inflammation and easing tension, Chamomile supports relief through softness and steady reassurance.

LEMON BALM
melissa officinalis

soften

HOW SHE MIGHT HELP

Pain intensified by stress, nervous system strain, or muscular guarding often responds well to Lemon Balm, especially when emotional and physical tension intertwine.

WORKING WITH HER

Gentle, consistent use allows Lemon Balm's calming and anti-inflammatory qualities to support comfort. She is most often taken as an infusion or tincture and fits well into routines that emphasize relaxation and recovery. Ongoing relationship supports ease and resilience.

AVOID COMBINING

Lemon Balm tends to feel most balanced when not layered heavily with other calming herbs used in high amounts. Thoughtful attention also serves those working with thyroid-related medications.

IMPORTANT NOTES

Lemon Balm suits ongoing use and is generally well tolerated. Beginning gently supports clear observation of the body's response, particularly when pain is closely tied to stress.

COMMON PREPARATIONS*

Tea (infusion)
Tincture

*See the Preparation Guide in the back of this book

WORKS WELL WITH

chamomile
skullcap
cleavers
turmeric
ginger

Through calming the nervous system and softening tension, Lemon Balm supports relief where pain is shaped by stress and holding.

WHITE WILLOW BARK
salix alba

HOW SHE MIGHT HELP

Persistent pain, inflammation, and discomfort linked to injury or chronic strain often respond to White Willow Bark, especially when more direct analgesic support is needed.

WORKING WITH HER

Measured, time-bound use allows White Willow Bark's pain-relieving qualities to support comfort. She is most often taken as a decoction, tincture, or capsule and fits well into routines addressing acute or ongoing inflammation. Thoughtful use supports relief without excess.

AVOID COMBINING

White Willow Bark tends to serve best when not layered with other salicylate-containing remedies or pharmaceutical pain relievers. Attentive use also supports those with sensitive digestion.

IMPORTANT NOTES

White Willow Bark carries a cooling, drying nature and suits short-term or targeted use. Careful attention supports those sensitive to aspirin-like compounds, and beginning gently allows the body's response to guide continued relationship.

---

ease

COMMON PREPARATIONS*

Tea (decoction)
Tincture
Capsule

*See the Preparation Guide in the back of this book

WORKS WELL WITH

turmeric
ginger
boswellia
skullcap
chamomile

By offering steady analgesic support, White Willow Bark helps ease pain and inflammation while allowing the body to remain engaged in repair.

SECTION FIVE

HORMONE & CYCLICAL SUPPORT

Hormonal health reflects the body's internal rhythms, shaping energy, mood, fertility, rest, and resilience across the lifespan. Cycles unfold through monthly patterns, seasonal shifts, and longer life stages, responding to nourishment, stress, movement, and rest. When hormonal systems feel supported, the body often settles into greater coherence and ease.

The remedies gathered here approach hormonal balance from many directions. Some nourish and steady foundational systems, supporting long-term regulation and adaptability. Others address specific moments within the cycle, easing discomfort, tension, or emotional fluctuation as they arise. Several work through the nervous system or circulatory pathways, illustrating how hormones respond to safety, rhythm, and relational support rather than forceful correction. Together, these plants reflect the interconnected nature of endocrine, emotional, and physical experience.

Roots, seeds, leaves, blossoms, and oils appear throughout these pages because of their long-standing use in supporting cyclical health across cultures and traditions. They demonstrate foundational hormonal patterns such as warming and cooling, building and moving, tonifying and releasing. Working with them reveals how balance emerges through consistency, timing, and attentiveness to change.

These pages invite an ongoing relationship with the body's cycles and signals. Attention to timing, sensation, and emotional tone becomes a form of listening guided by plants that have long supported reproductive health, transition, and renewal. May this collection offer a steady entry point into hormonal care and deepen understanding of the rhythms that shape vitality across seasons and stages of life.

wild yam root
kudzu root
maca root
red clover
fenugreek
ashwagandha
vitex
black cohosh
dong quai
shatavari
eve. primrose
white peony
motherwort
red raspberry
cramp bark
yarrow
mugwort
ginger

WILD YAM ROOT
dioscorea villosa

ease

HOW SHE MIGHT HELP
Cyclical discomfort, cramping, and tension linked to hormonal shifts often soften with Wild Yam, especially when the body seeks relaxation and gentle regulation.

WORKING WITH HER
Consistent, attentive use allows Wild Yam's antispasmodic qualities to support ease across the cycle. She is most often taken as a tincture or decoction and fits well into routines focused on calming muscular tension and supporting hormonal comfort. Ongoing relationship supports steadiness and relief.

AVOID COMBINING
Wild Yam integrates smoothly with many hormone-supportive herbs. Thoughtful pacing supports balance when layering with strongly sedative remedies used in high amounts.

IMPORTANT NOTES
Wild Yam suits moderate, ongoing use and is generally well tolerated. Beginning gently supports clear awareness of the body's response as patterns unfold.

COMMON PREPARATIONS*

Tincture
Tea (decoction)

*See the Preparation Guide in the back of this book

WORKS WELL WITH

cramp bark
black cohosh
motherwort
ginger
chamomile

By easing tension and calming spasm, Wild Yam supports the body in moving through hormonal shifts with greater comfort.

KUDZU ROOT
pueraria lobata

cool

HOW SHE MIGHT HELP

Hormonal fluctuation, heat, and discomfort linked to transition often respond well to Kudzu, especially when cooling and nourishing support benefits balance.

WORKING WITH HER

Steady, patient use allows Kudzu's soothing qualities to support hormonal equilibrium over time. She is most often taken as a decoction, tincture, or powder and fits well into routines addressing transition and cyclical change. Ongoing relationship supports steadiness and ease.

AVOID COMBINING

Kudzu tends to serve best alongside gentle hormone-supportive herbs. Attentive use supports comfort when layering with strong phytoestrogenic remedies used in high amounts.

IMPORTANT NOTES

Kudzu offers a cooling, moistening profile and suits consistent use. Beginning gently supports observation of the body's response, particularly during periods of heat or transition.

COMMON PREPARATIONS*

Tea (decoction)
Tincture
Powder

*See the Preparation Guide in the back of this book

WORKS WELL WITH

red clover blossoms
dong quai
white peony
maca root
ginger

Through cooling nourishment and steady support, Kudzu helps the body find balance during hormonal transition.

MACA ROOT POWDER
lepidium meyenii

nourish

HOW SHE MIGHT HELP
Low energy, hormonal fatigue, and reduced resilience across the cycle often benefit from Maca, especially when vitality and adaptability need support.

WORKING WITH HER
Regular, consistent use allows Maca's nourishing qualities to build gradually. She is most often taken as a powder blended into food or drink and fits well into daily routines focused on hormonal stamina and balance. Ongoing relationship supports strength and endurance.

AVOID COMBINING
Maca integrates smoothly with many hormone-supportive herbs. Thoughtful pacing supports balance when layering with strong stimulating tonics used in high amounts.

IMPORTANT NOTES
Maca carries a warming, energizing nature and suits measured use. Beginning gently supports awareness of the body's response, particularly during the first weeks of use.

COMMON PREPARATIONS*

Powder

*See the Preparation Guide in the back of this book

WORKS WELL WITH
ashwagandha root
shatavari
red clover blossoms
white peony
ginger

By nourishing energy and adaptability, Maca supports hormonal resilience across changing cycles.

RED CLOVER BLOSSOMS
trifolium pratense

cool

HOW SHE MIGHT HELP

Hormonal imbalance, heat, and cyclical discomfort often ease with Red Clover, especially when gentle cleansing and cooling support benefit balance.

WORKING WITH HER

Steady, long-view use allows Red Clover's nourishing qualities to support hormonal equilibrium. She is most often taken as an infusion or tincture and fits well into routines focused on gradual balance and transition. Ongoing relationship supports ease and clarity.

AVOID COMBINING

Red Clover generally integrates smoothly with a wide range of hormone-supportive herbs. Attentive use supports comfort when layering with concentrated phytoestrogenic remedies used in high amounts.

IMPORTANT NOTES

Red Clover offers a cooling, cleansing profile and suits consistent use. Beginning gently supports observation of the body's response over time.

COMMON PREPARATIONS*

Tea (infusion)
Tincture

*See the Preparation Guide in the back of this book

WORKS WELL WITH

kudzu root
white peony
dong quai
shatavari
maca root

Through gentle nourishment and cleansing support, Red Clover helps the body settle into hormonal balance with ease.

FENUGREEK
trigonella foenum-graecum

energy

HOW SHE MIGHT HELP

Hormonal depletion, low vitality, and dryness across the cycle often respond well to Fenugreek, especially when nourishment and rebuilding support are needed.

WORKING WITH HER

Steady, intentional use allows Fenugreek's warming and nutritive qualities to support hormonal balance. She is most often taken as a decoction, powder, or tincture and fits well into routines focused on restoration and strength. Ongoing relationship supports grounded energy and comfort.

AVOID COMBINING

Fenugreek tends to feel most balanced when not layered heavily with other strongly warming or stimulating herbs used in high amounts. Thoughtful attention also supports those sensitive to blood sugar shifts.

IMPORTANT NOTES

Fenugreek carries a warming, moistening nature and suits moderate, consistent use. Beginning gently supports awareness of the body's response, particularly for digestion and metabolism.

COMMON PREPARATIONS*

Tea (decoction)
Tincture
Powder

*See the Preparation Guide in the back of this book

WORKS WELL WITH

shatavari
maca root
ginger
red raspberry leaf
ashwagandha

By nourishing and rebuilding from within, Fenugreek supports hormonal strength and sustained vitality.

ASHWAGANDHA ROOT POWDER
withania somnifera

restore

HOW SHE MIGHT HELP

Hormonal fatigue, stress-related imbalance, and nervous system depletion often soften with Ashwagandha, especially when cycles feel strained by ongoing demand.

WORKING WITH HER

Consistent, long-view use allows Ashwagandha's grounding qualities to support endocrine balance. She is most often taken as a powder blended into food or drink and fits well into daily routines focused on steadiness and restoration. Ongoing relationship supports resilience across cycles.

AVOID COMBINING

Ashwagandha tends to serve best when not layered with other strong stimulating adaptogens used in high amounts. Attentive use also supports those working with thyroid-related medications.

IMPORTANT NOTES

Ashwagandha offers deep, restorative support and suits steady rather than short-term use. Beginning gently supports clear observation of the body's response as balance unfolds.

COMMON PREPARATIONS*

Powder
Capsule
Tincture

*See the Preparation Guide in the back of this book

WORKS WELL WITH

shatavari
maca root
vitex
ginger
red raspberry leaf

Through grounding and restoration, Ashwagandha supports hormonal balance by strengthening resilience under stress.

VITEX (CHASTEBERRY)

vitex agnus-castus

regulate

HOW SHE MIGHT HELP

Irregular cycles, cyclical discomfort, and hormonal imbalance often benefit from Vitex, especially when rhythm and regulation need steady support.

WORKING WITH HER

Patient, consistent use allows Vitex's regulatory qualities to influence the hormonal cycle over time. She is most often taken as a tincture or capsule and fits well into routines focused on long-term balance rather than immediate relief. Ongoing relationship supports clearer cyclical patterns.

AVOID COMBINING

Vitex tends to serve best when used on her own rather than layered with multiple hormone-regulating remedies. Thoughtful attention also supports those working with hormonal medications.

IMPORTANT NOTES

Vitex works gradually and suits extended use. Beginning gently supports awareness of the body's response, particularly across several cycles.

COMMON PREPARATIONS*

Tincture
Capsule

*See the Preparation Guide in the back of this book

WORKS WELL WITH

red raspberry leaf
white peony
dong quai
ashwagandha
motherwort

By supporting hormonal rhythm and timing, Vitex helps the body reestablish clarity and balance across the cycle.

BLACK COHOSH
actaea racemosa

steady

HOW SHE MIGHT HELP

Intense cyclical transitions, heat, and discomfort linked to hormonal shifts often ease with Black Cohosh, especially when the body seeks grounding and relief through change.

WORKING WITH HER

Measured, intentional use allows Black Cohosh's regulating qualities to support the nervous and hormonal systems together. She is most often taken as a tincture or capsule and fits well into routines focused on transitional support rather than daily nourishment. Thoughtful relationship supports steadiness through change.

AVOID COMBINING

Black Cohosh tends to serve best when not layered heavily with other strong hormone-regulating remedies. Attentive use supports balance when combining with long-term endocrine tonics.

IMPORTANT NOTES

Black Cohosh carries a focused, downward-moving nature and suits time-bound use. Beginning gently supports awareness of the body's response, particularly during periods of significant hormonal transition.

COMMON PREPARATIONS*

Tincture
Capsule

*See the Preparation Guide in the back of this book

WORKS WELL WITH

dong quai
vitex
motherwort
red clover blossoms

Through deep grounding and nervous system support, Black Cohosh helps the body move through hormonal transition with greater steadiness.

DONG QUAI
angelica sinensis

balance

HOW SHE MIGHT HELP

Cyclical irregularity, blood stagnation, and discomfort often benefit from Dong Quai, especially when circulation and nourishment support hormonal balance.

WORKING WITH HER

Steady, consistent use allows Dong Quai's harmonizing qualities to support the reproductive system over time. She is most often taken as a decoction, tincture, or capsule and fits well into routines focused on long-view cyclical regulation. Ongoing relationship supports flow and balance.

AVOID COMBINING

Dong Quai tends to feel most balanced when not layered heavily with strong blood-moving or anticoagulant remedies. Thoughtful attention supports comfort when combining with warming circulatory herbs.

IMPORTANT NOTES

Dong Quai offers warming, circulatory support and suits moderate use. Beginning gently supports observation of the body's response, particularly during changes in cycle length or flow.

COMMON PREPARATIONS*

Tea (decoction)
Tincture
Capsule

*See the Preparation Guide in the back of this book

WORKS WELL WITH

white peony
red clover blossoms
vitex
shatavari
ginger

By supporting circulation and nourishment, Dong Quai helps restore rhythm and ease across the menstrual cycle.

SHATAVARI
asparagus racemosus

restore

HOW SHE MIGHT HELP

Dryness, depletion, and hormonal fatigue often soften with Shatavari, especially when the body benefits from deep nourishment and replenishment.

WORKING WITH HER

Gentle, consistent use allows Shatavari's rebuilding qualities to support endocrine balance over time. She is most often taken as a powder or tincture and fits well into routines focused on restoration and long-term support. Ongoing relationship supports softness and resilience.

AVOID COMBINING

Shatavari integrates smoothly with many hormone-supportive herbs. Attentive use supports balance when layering with strongly stimulating tonics used in high amounts.

IMPORTANT NOTES

Shatavari carries a cooling, moistening nature and suits ongoing use. Beginning gently supports awareness of the body's response, particularly during periods of depletion.

COMMON PREPARATIONS*

Powder
Tincture

*See the Preparation Guide in the back of this book

WORKS WELL WITH

ashwagandha
maca root
red clover blossoms
white peony
fenugreek

Through deep nourishment and restoration, Shatavari supports hormonal balance and sustained vitality.

EVENING PRIMROSE
oenothera biennis

support

HOW SHE MIGHT HELP

Cyclical discomfort, breast tenderness, and inflammation linked to hormonal fluctuation often respond well to Evening Primrose, especially when tissue support and balance are needed.

WORKING WITH HER

Regular, steady use allows Evening Primrose's fatty acid profile to support hormonal and inflammatory balance. She is most often taken as an oil in capsule form and fits well into routines focused on cyclical comfort. Ongoing relationship supports ease across the cycle.

AVOID COMBINING

Evening Primrose generally integrates smoothly with many hormone-supportive remedies. Thoughtful attention supports balance when layering with other concentrated fatty acid supplements.

IMPORTANT NOTES

Evening Primrose suits consistent use and is typically well tolerated. Beginning gently supports awareness of the body's response, particularly during the luteal phase.

COMMON PREPARATIONS*

Capsule (oil)

*See the Preparation Guide in the back of this book

WORKS WELL WITH

vitex
red raspberry leaf
shatavari
chamomile
lemon balm

By supporting tissue health and inflammatory balance, Evening Primrose helps ease cyclical discomfort and promote hormonal harmony.

WHITE PEONY
paeonia lactiflora

soften

HOW SHE MIGHT HELP

Cyclical tension, hormonal imbalance, and discomfort linked to constraint or stagnation often respond well to White Peony, especially when softness and regulation support ease.

WORKING WITH HER

Steady, consistent use allows White Peony's harmonizing qualities to support balance across the cycle. She is most often taken as a decoction or tincture and fits well into routines focused on smoothing hormonal patterns over time. Ongoing relationship supports flexibility and relief.

AVOID COMBINING

White Peony tends to serve best when not layered heavily with other strong blood-moving or hormone-regulating remedies. Thoughtful attention supports comfort when combining with warming circulatory herbs.

IMPORTANT NOTES

White Peony carries a cooling, softening nature and suits moderate, ongoing use. Beginning gently supports awareness of the body's response, particularly during periods of tension or imbalance.

COMMON PREPARATIONS*

Tea (decoction)
Tincture

*See the Preparation Guide in the back of this book

WORKS WELL WITH

dong quai
shatavari
vitex
red clover blossoms
ginger

Through softening and regulation, White Peony supports the body in finding ease within hormonal rhythm.

MOTHERWORT
leonurus cardiaca

steady

HOW SHE MIGHT HELP

Emotional intensity, cyclical anxiety, and heart-centered tension often ease with Motherwort, especially when stress and hormonal shifts intersect.

WORKING WITH HER

Gentle, attentive use allows Motherwort's steadying qualities to support both emotional and hormonal balance. She is most often taken as a tincture or infusion and fits well into routines that emphasize calming and grounding through change. Ongoing relationship supports reassurance and ease.

AVOID COMBINING

Motherwort tends to feel most balanced when not layered heavily with other strong sedative remedies used in high amounts. Thoughtful attention also serves those working with heart-related medications.

IMPORTANT NOTES

Motherwort suits moderate, ongoing use and is generally well tolerated. Beginning gently supports clear observation of the body's response, particularly when emotional patterns are closely tied to the cycle.

COMMON PREPARATIONS*

Tincture
Tea (infusion)

*See the Preparation Guide in the back of this book

WORKS WELL WITH

vitex
wild yam root
white peony
lemon balm
chamomile

By calming the heart and steadying emotional response, Motherwort supports balance through hormonal transition.

RED RASPBERRY LEAF
rubus idaeus

support

HOW SHE MIGHT HELP

Cyclical weakness, uterine fatigue, and discomfort linked to tone and endurance often benefit from Red Raspberry Leaf, especially when gentle strengthening supports balance.

WORKING WITH HER

Consistent, long-view use allows Red Raspberry Leaf's tonifying qualities to support uterine health and cyclical resilience. She is most often taken as an infusion and fits well into daily routines focused on steady support. Ongoing relationship supports strength and reliability across the cycle.

AVOID COMBINING

Red Raspberry Leaf generally integrates smoothly with many hormone-supportive herbs. Attentive use supports balance when layering with strongly astringent remedies used in high amounts.

IMPORTANT NOTES

Red Raspberry Leaf suits ongoing use and is typically well tolerated. Beginning gently supports awareness of the body's response, particularly during long-term cycle support.

COMMON PREPARATIONS*

Tea (infusion)
Tincture

*See the Preparation Guide in the back of this book

WORKS WELL WITH

vitex
evening primrose
cramp bark
shatavari
ginger

Through steady toning and nourishment, Red Raspberry Leaf supports strength and continuity within the menstrual cycle.

CRAMPBARK
viburnum opulus

ease

HOW SHE MIGHT HELP

Painful cramping, muscular spasm, and cyclical tension often soften with Cramp Bark, especially when the body benefits from release and relaxation.

WORKING WITH HER

Targeted, attentive use allows Cramp Bark's antispasmodic qualities to support comfort during acute cyclical discomfort. She is most often taken as a tincture or decoction and fits well into routines focused on relief during active cramping. Thoughtful use supports ease without dulling awareness.

AVOID COMBINING

Cramp Bark tends to serve best when not layered heavily with other strong sedative or antispasmodic remedies used in high amounts. Attentive pacing supports clarity of effect.

IMPORTANT NOTES

Cramp Bark suits short-term or cyclical use rather than daily support. Beginning gently supports clear observation of the body's response, particularly during periods of acute discomfort.

COMMON PREPARATIONS*

Tincture
Tea (decoction)

*See the Preparation Guide in the back of this book

WORKS WELL WITH

wild yam root
red raspberry leaf
motherwort
ginger
chamomile

By easing spasm and restoring calm to the muscles, Cramp Bark supports relief during the most intense moments of the cycle.

YARROW
achillea millefolium

flow

HOW SHE MIGHT HELP

Irregular flow, cyclical tension, and discomfort shaped by stagnation often respond to Yarrow, especially when gentle movement and balance support the body's rhythm.

WORKING WITH HER

Attentive, moderate use allows Yarrow's regulating qualities to support circulation and ease across the cycle. She is most often taken as an infusion or tincture and fits well into routines focused on restoring flow without excess stimulation. Ongoing relationship supports steadiness and clarity.

AVOID COMBINING

Yarrow tends to feel most balanced when not layered heavily with other strong blood-moving remedies used in high amounts. Thoughtful pacing supports comfort when combining with astringent or drying herbs.

IMPORTANT NOTES

Yarrow carries a drying, regulating nature and suits measured use. Beginning gently supports awareness of the body's response, particularly during shifts in flow or cycle intensity.

COMMON PREPARATIONS*

Tea (infusion)
Tincture

*See the Preparation Guide in the back of this book

WORKS WELL WITH

red raspberry leaf
white peony
ginger
motherwort
vitex

By supporting balanced movement and flow, Yarrow helps the body find steadiness within cyclical change.

MUGWORT
artemisia vulgaris

attune

HOW SHE MIGHT HELP

Disrupted cycles, delayed flow, and patterns shaped by stagnation or disconnection often respond to Mugwort, especially when rhythm and awareness benefit from gentle encouragement.

WORKING WITH HER

Intentional, time-aware use allows Mugwort's moving and warming qualities to support cyclical regulation. She is most often taken as an infusion, tincture, or used ceremonially and fits well into practices focused on reconnecting with timing and bodily awareness. Thoughtful relationship supports clarity and flow.

AVOID COMBINING

Mugwort tends to serve best when not layered heavily with other strong emmenagogues or intensely stimulating remedies. Attentive pacing supports balance, particularly when working close to the cycle.

IMPORTANT NOTES

Mugwort carries a warming, activating nature and suits measured use. She is traditionally avoided during pregnancy, and beginning gently supports clear observation of the body's response.

COMMON PREPARATIONS*

Tea (infusion)
Tincture
Topical or ceremonial use

*See the Preparation Guide in the back of this book

WORKS WELL WITH

yarrow
ginger
motherwort
white peony
red raspberry leaf

By supporting rhythm and embodied awareness, Mugwort helps restore connection to the body's natural timing.

GINGER
zingiber officinale

warm

HOW SHE MIGHT HELP
Cold, stagnation, and cyclical discomfort often ease with Ginger, especially when warmth and circulation support comfort and regularity.

WORKING WITH HER
Consistent, moderate use allows Ginger's warming qualities to support movement and ease across the cycle. She is most often taken as an infusion, decoction, powder, or tincture and fits well into routines focused on relieving tension and supporting flow. Ongoing relationship supports steadiness and comfort.

AVOID COMBINING
Ginger tends to feel most balanced when not layered heavily with other strongly heating remedies used in high amounts. Thoughtful attention supports comfort for those sensitive to warmth.

IMPORTANT NOTES
Ginger carries an activating, warming nature and suits measured use. Beginning gently supports awareness of the body's response, particularly during periods of heat or intensity.

COMMON PREPARATIONS*

Tea (infusion or decoction)
Powder
Tincture
Food-based preparations

*See the Preparation Guide in the back of this book

WORKS WELL WITH

cramp bark
dong quai
vitex
red raspberry leaf
maca root

Through warmth and circulation, Ginger helps integrate and support hormonal flow across the cycle

SECTION SIX
ENERGY, MOOD & VITALITY

Vitality reflects how the body meets daily life with presence, resilience, and clarity. Energy moves through physical stamina, emotional tone, focus, and motivation, shaped by nourishment, stress, rest, and rhythm. When these systems feel supported, vitality often expresses itself as steadiness rather than force and endurance rather than urgency.

The remedies gathered here support energy and mood through multiple pathways. Some nourish foundational reserves, helping rebuild strength after depletion or prolonged demand. Others sharpen clarity, uplift emotional tone, or support adaptive response during periods of stress and change. Several work through the nervous system and circulatory pathways, illustrating how vitality emerges from balance, safety, and steady engagement rather than stimulation alone.

Roots, leaves, berries, and tonics appear throughout these pages because of their long-standing role in supporting stamina and emotional resilience across cultures and traditions. Together, they demonstrate core vitality patterns such as building and activating, calming and focusing, grounding and uplifting. Working with them reveals how energy responds to consistency, timing, and thoughtful pacing.

These pages invite attentiveness to how energy rises, settles, and renews throughout the day and across seasons. Observing mood, motivation, and capacity becomes a form of listening, guided by plants that have long supported sustainable vitality and clear presence. May this collection offer a steady entry point into energy and mood support and deepen understanding of the rhythms that allow vitality to endure.

schisandra
maca root
kudzu root
ashwagandha
rhodiola root
tulsi
gotu kola
lemon balm
peppermint
yerba mate
eleuthero

SCHISANDRA BERRIES
schisandra chinensis

focus

HOW SHE MIGHT HELP
Fluctuating energy, stress-related fatigue, and difficulty sustaining focus often respond well to Schisandra, especially when stamina and emotional steadiness need support together.

WORKING WITH HER
Consistent, intentional use allows Schisandra's adaptogenic qualities to support resilience across physical and emotional systems. She is most often taken as a tincture, decoction, or powder and fits well into routines focused on steady energy and mental clarity. Ongoing relationship supports endurance without depletion.

AVOID COMBINING
Schisandra tends to feel most balanced when not layered heavily with multiple stimulating adaptogens used at the same time. Thoughtful pacing supports clarity when combining with energizing tonics.

IMPORTANT NOTES
Schisandra carries a focused, tonifying nature and suits ongoing use. Beginning gently supports awareness of the body's response, particularly in digestion and sleep.

COMMON PREPARATIONS*

Tea (decoction)
Tincture
Powder

*See the Preparation Guide in the back of this book

WORKS WELL WITH

eleuthero
ashwagandha
tulsi
gotu kola
lemon balm

By supporting adaptability and focus, Schisandra helps energy remain steady under sustained demand.

MACA ROOT
lepidium meyenii

nourish

HOW SHE MIGHT HELP
Low stamina, diminished motivation, and hormonal-related fatigue often benefit from Maca, especially when the body seeks nourishment and renewed vitality.

WORKING WITH HER
Regular, steady use allows Maca's nutritive qualities to build gradually. She is most often taken as a powder blended into food or drink and fits well into daily routines focused on sustained energy and resilience. Ongoing relationship supports strength without overstimulation.

AVOID COMBINING
Maca generally integrates smoothly with many vitality-supportive herbs. Thoughtful attention supports balance when layering with strongly stimulating tonics used in high amounts.

IMPORTANT NOTES
Maca carries a warming, strengthening nature and suits measured use. Beginning gently supports awareness of the body's response, particularly during the first weeks of use.

COMMON PREPARATIONS*

Powder

*See the Preparation Guide in the back of this book

WORKS WELL WITH
ashwagandha
schisandra berries
tulsi
gotu kola
lemon balm

Through nourishment and stamina-building support, Maca helps restore vitality and motivation.

KUDZU ROOT
pueraria lobata

calm

HOW SHE MIGHT HELP

Energy depletion paired with tension, heat, or stress-related imbalance often softens with Kudzu, especially when steadiness and cooling support are needed.

WORKING WITH HER

Steady, patient use allows Kudzu's grounding qualities to support calm energy and emotional balance. She is most often taken as a decoction, tincture, or powder and fits well into routines focused on smoothing fluctuations rather than pushing output. Ongoing relationship supports ease.

AVOID COMBINING

Kudzu tends to serve best when not layered heavily with multiple phytoestrogenic or strongly tonifying remedies used in high amounts. Attentive pacing supports balance.

IMPORTANT NOTES

Kudzu offers a cooling, moistening profile and suits consistent use. Beginning gently supports clear observation of the body's response during periods of stress or transition.

COMMON PREPARATIONS*

Tea (decoction)
Tincture
Powder

*See the Preparation Guide in the back of this book

WORKS WELL WITH

lemon balm
ashwagandha
schisandra berries
gotu kola
tulsi

By calming excess strain and supporting steady output, Kudzu helps energy settle into balance.

ASHWAGANDHA ROOT
withania somnifera

restore

HOW SHE MIGHT HELP

Chronic stress, nervous exhaustion, and depleted vitality often respond to Ashwagandha, especially when energy feels drained by ongoing demand.

WORKING WITH HER

Consistent, long-view use allows Ashwagandha's grounding qualities to support both energy and mood. She is most often taken as a powder, tincture, or capsule and fits well into routines focused on restoration rather than stimulation. Ongoing relationship supports resilience and steadiness.

AVOID COMBINING

Ashwagandha tends to serve best when not layered heavily with strongly stimulating adaptogens used at the same time. Thoughtful attention also supports those working with thyroid-related medications.

IMPORTANT NOTES

Ashwagandha suits steady, ongoing use rather than short-term energy boosting. Beginning gently supports awareness of the body's response as balance returns.

COMMON PREPARATIONS*

Powder
Tincture
Capsule

*See the Preparation Guide in the back of this book

WORKS WELL WITH

maca root
schisandra berries
tulsi
lemon balm
gotu kola

Through restoration and nervous system support, Ashwagandha helps vitality rebuild from a stable foundation.

RHODIOLA ROOT
rhodiola rosea

stimulate

HOW SHE MIGHT HELP

Mental fatigue, low motivation, and stress-related burnout often respond well to Rhodiola, especially when clarity and endurance feel diminished by ongoing pressure.

WORKING WITH HER

Intentional, time-aware use allows Rhodiola's stimulating adaptogenic qualities to support alertness and emotional resilience. She is most often taken as a tincture or capsule and fits well into morning routines that benefit from focused energy and mental stamina. Thoughtful relationship supports engagement without depletion.

AVOID COMBINING

Rhodiola tends to serve best when not layered with other strongly stimulating adaptogens used at the same time. Attentive pacing supports balance when working with caffeine or activating tonics.

IMPORTANT NOTES

Rhodiola carries an uplifting, activating nature and suits measured use. Beginning gently supports awareness of the body's response, particularly in sleep and nervous system tone.

COMMON PREPARATIONS*

Tincture
Capsule

*See the Preparation Guide in the back of this book

WORKS WELL WITH

schisandra berries
eleuthero
tulsi
lemon balm
gotu kola

By supporting clarity and endurance, Rhodiola helps energy rise with focus and intention.

TULSI
(HOLY BASIL)

ocimum tenuiflorum

calm

HOW SHE MIGHT HELP

Emotional strain, stress-related fatigue, and mood fluctuation often soften with Tulsi, especially when vitality benefits from calm uplift rather than stimulation.

WORKING WITH HER

Consistent, gentle use allows Tulsi's balancing qualities to support both energy and emotional steadiness. She is most often taken as an infusion or tincture and fits well into daily routines focused on resilience and clarity. Ongoing relationship supports grounded vitality.

AVOID COMBINING

Tulsi generally integrates smoothly with many adaptogenic herbs. Thoughtful attention supports balance when layering with strong stimulants used in high amounts.

IMPORTANT NOTES

Tulsi carries a warming, clarifying nature and suits ongoing use. Beginning gently supports observation of the body's response across mood and energy patterns.

COMMON PREPARATIONS*

Tea (infusion)
Tincture

*See the Preparation Guide in the back of this book

WORKS WELL WITH

ashwagandha
schisandra berries
lemon balm
gotu kola
maca root

Through calm uplift and steady presence, Tulsi supports vitality rooted in balance.

GOTU KOLA
centella asiatica

clarify

HOW SHE MIGHT HELP

Mental fog, scattered focus, and nervous fatigue often respond well to Gotu Kola, especially when clarity and grounded energy need support together.

WORKING WITH HER

Gentle, consistent use allows Gotu Kola's centering qualities to support cognitive function and emotional steadiness. She is most often taken as an infusion or tincture and fits well into routines focused on focus without overstimulation. Ongoing relationship supports clarity and calm engagement.

AVOID COMBINING

Gotu Kola tends to feel most balanced when not layered heavily with strong sedatives or intense stimulants. Attentive pacing supports clarity of effect.

IMPORTANT NOTES

Gotu Kola offers cooling, grounding support and suits moderate use. Beginning gently supports awareness of the body's response, particularly in mood and concentration.

COMMON PREPARATIONS*

Tea (infusion)
Tincture

*See the Preparation Guide in the back of this book

WORKS WELL WITH

lemon balm
tulsi (holy basil)
schisandra berries
oatstraw
ashwagandha

Traditionally valued for supporting clarity, circulation, and steady renewal, Gotu Kola encourages balanced energy that feels grounded, focused, and sustained.

LEMON BALM
melissa officinalis

ease

HOW SHE MIGHT HELP

Low mood, nervous tension, and energy shaped by stress often ease with Lemon Balm, especially when emotional comfort and gentle uplift support vitality.

WORKING WITH HER

Consistent, soothing use allows Lemon Balm's calming qualities to support mood and nervous system balance. She is most often taken as an infusion or tincture and fits well into routines focused on emotional steadiness and ease. Ongoing relationship supports gentle renewal.

AVOID COMBINING

Lemon Balm tends to feel most balanced when not layered heavily with other calming herbs used in high amounts. Thoughtful attention also serves those working with thyroid-related medications.

IMPORTANT NOTES

Lemon Balm suits ongoing use and is generally well tolerated. Beginning gently supports clear observation of the body's response across mood and energy.

COMMON PREPARATIONS*

Tea (infusion)
Tincture

*See the Preparation Guide in the back of this book

WORKS WELL WITH

tulsi
gotu kola
schisandra berries
peppermint
ashwagandha

Through calm reassurance and gentle uplift, Lemon Balm supports vitality shaped by emotional ease.

PEPPERMINT
mentha x piperita

energize

HOW SHE MIGHT HELP

Mental sluggishness, low motivation, and energy weighed down by tension often lift with Peppermint, especially when clarity and gentle stimulation support renewed focus.

WORKING WITH HER

Light, intentional use allows Peppermint's brightening qualities to support alertness and mood. She is most often taken as an infusion or tincture and fits well into routines that benefit from quick clarity and refreshed attention. Thoughtful relationship supports engagement without overwhelm.

AVOID COMBINING

Peppermint tends to feel most balanced when not layered heavily with other strongly stimulating herbs used in high amounts. Attentive pacing supports comfort for those sensitive to cooling or activation.

IMPORTANT NOTES

Peppermint carries a cooling, dispersing nature and suits moderate use. Beginning gently supports awareness of the body's response, particularly in digestion and nervous system tone.

COMMON PREPARATIONS*

Tea (infusion)
Tincture

*See the Preparation Guide in the back of this book

WORKS WELL WITH

lemon balm
gotu kola
tulsi
schisandra berries
yerba mate

Through clarity and lift, Peppermint helps energy feel lighter and more accessible.

YERBA MATE
ilex paraguariensis

stamina

HOW SHE MIGHT HELP
Fatigue, low drive, and diminished alertness often respond to Yerba Mate, especially when sustained energy and mental engagement are needed.

WORKING WITH HER
Mindful, time-aware use allows Yerba Mate's stimulating qualities to support stamina and focus. She is most often taken as an infusion and fits well into morning or early-day routines that call for clear, steady energy. Thoughtful relationship supports vitality without excess strain.

AVOID COMBINING
Yerba Mate tends to serve best when not layered heavily with other caffeinated or strongly stimulating remedies. Attentive pacing supports balance when working with activating adaptogens.

IMPORTANT NOTES
Yerba Mate carries an activating nature and suits measured use. Beginning gently supports awareness of the body's response, particularly in sleep and nervous system tone.

COMMON PREPARATIONS*

Tea (infusion)

*See the Preparation Guide in the back of this book

WORKS WELL WITH
peppermint
tulsi
schisandra berries
eleuthero
lemon balm

By supporting alert presence and sustained stamina, Yerba Mate helps energy remain engaged and clear.

ELEUTHERO
eleutherococcus senticosus

revitalize

HOW SHE MIGHT HELP

Stress-related fatigue, depleted reserves, and difficulty sustaining effort often benefit from Eleuthero, especially when adaptability and endurance need reinforcement.

WORKING WITH HER

Consistent, long-view use allows Eleuthero's adaptogenic qualities to strengthen resilience over time. She is most often taken as a tincture, capsule, or decoction and fits well into routines focused on steady stamina rather than quick stimulation. Ongoing relationship supports durability and balance.

AVOID COMBINING

Eleuthero tends to feel most balanced when not layered heavily with other strongly stimulating adaptogens used at the same time. Thoughtful pacing supports clarity of effect.

IMPORTANT NOTES

Eleuthero carries a strengthening, neutral nature and suits ongoing use. Beginning gently supports awareness of the body's response as stamina builds.

COMMON PREPARATIONS*

Tea (decoction)
Tincture
Capsule

*See the Preparation Guide in the back of this book

WORKS WELL WITH

schisandra berries
rhodiola
tulsi
ashwagandha
yerba mate

Through steady adaptive support, Eleuthero helps vitality endure across sustained demand.

SECTION SEVEN
CIRCULATION & HEART SUPPORT

Circulation reflects how the body moves life force, nourishment, and warmth through every tissue. The heart and vascular system respond continuously to movement, emotion, stress, and rest, shaping vitality, endurance, and emotional resilience. When circulation feels supported, the body often experiences greater ease, warmth, and coherence.

The remedies gathered here support circulatory and heart health through a wide range of actions. Some strengthen and nourish the heart itself, supporting rhythm and long-term resilience. Others encourage movement, helping ease stagnation and restore flow through vessels and tissues. Several address the emotional dimensions of the heart, illustrating how circulation responds to calm, reassurance, and steady presence as much as physical activity. Together, these plants reflect the intimate relationship between circulation, vitality, and emotional tone.

Berries, leaves, roots, flowers, and warming spices appear throughout these pages because of their long-standing use across cultures and traditions. They demonstrate foundational circulatory patterns such as building and moving, warming and toning, relaxing and strengthening. Working with them reveals how circulation responds to consistency, balance, and thoughtful engagement rather than force.

These pages invite awareness of warmth, pulse, breath, and emotional steadiness. Attention to how energy moves through the body becomes a form of listening, guided by plants that have long supported heart health and healthy circulation. May this collection offer a steady entry point into circulatory care and deepen understanding of the relationships that allow the heart and vessels to function with strength and grace.

hawthorn
motherwort
rose petals
hibiscus flower
ginger
turmeric
cayenne
garlic
ginkgo
yarrow
schisandra
red sage root
rosemary

HAWTHORN BERRY
crataegus monogyna

HOW SHE MIGHT HELP
Long-term heart support, circulatory weakness, and fatigue linked to endurance often respond well to Hawthorn Berry, especially when nourishment and strengthening are needed together.

WORKING WITH HER
Consistent, patient use allows Hawthorn Berry's nourishing qualities to support cardiovascular resilience over time. She is most often taken as a tincture, decoction, or capsule and fits well into routines focused on steady heart support. Ongoing relationship supports strength and reliability.

AVOID COMBINING
Hawthorn Berry generally integrates smoothly with many circulatory herbs. Thoughtful attention supports balance when layering with concentrated cardiovascular supplements.

IMPORTANT NOTES
Hawthorn Berry suits long-term, ongoing use and is typically well tolerated. Beginning gently supports awareness of the body's response, particularly during extended heart-focused routines.

---

nourish

COMMON PREPARATIONS*

Tea (decoction)
Tincture
Capsule

*See the Preparation Guide in the back of this book

WORKS WELL WITH

hawthorn leaf and flower
rose petals
motherwort
schisandra berries
ginkgo

Through steady nourishment and strengthening, Hawthorn Berry supports the heart in maintaining endurance and balance.

HAWTHORN LEAF & FLOWER
crataegus monogyna

calm

HOW SHE MIGHT HELP

Circulatory tension, emotional strain, and fluctuations in heart rhythm often ease with Hawthorn Leaf and Flower, especially when calming and toning support are needed together.

WORKING WITH HER

Gentle, consistent use allows Hawthorn Leaf and Flower's balancing qualities to support both circulation and emotional steadiness. She is most often taken as an infusion or tincture and fits well into routines focused on relaxation and heart-centered support. Ongoing relationship supports coherence and ease.

AVOID COMBINING

Hawthorn Leaf and Flower generally integrate smoothly with many heart-supportive herbs. Attentive pacing supports comfort when layering with strong circulatory stimulants.

IMPORTANT NOTES

Hawthorn Leaf and Flower suit ongoing use and are typically well tolerated. Beginning gently supports observation of the body's response across emotional and physical heart patterns.

COMMON PREPARATIONS*

Tea (infusion)
Tincture

*See the Preparation Guide in the back of this book

WORKS WELL WITH

hawthorn berry
motherwort
rose petals
lemon balm
yarrow

By calming and toning the heart, Hawthorn Leaf and Flower support circulation shaped by steadiness and ease.

MOTHERWORT
leonurus cardiaca

steady

HOW SHE MIGHT HELP

Heart-centered tension, emotional overwhelm, and circulatory strain often soften with Motherwort, especially when stress and heart rhythm feel closely linked.

WORKING WITH HER

Gentle, attentive use allows Motherwort's calming qualities to support emotional regulation and circulatory balance. She is most often taken as a tincture or infusion and fits well into routines focused on reassurance and grounding. Ongoing relationship supports steadiness through change.

AVOID COMBINING

Motherwort tends to feel most balanced when not layered heavily with other strong sedative remedies used in high amounts. Thoughtful attention also serves those working with heart-related medications.

IMPORTANT NOTES

Motherwort suits moderate, ongoing use and is generally well tolerated. Beginning gently supports awareness of the body's response, particularly during periods of emotional strain.

COMMON PREPARATIONS*

Tincture
Tea (infusion)

*See the Preparation Guide in the back of this book

WORKS WELL WITH

hawthorn leaf and flower
rose petals
lemon balm
yarrow
schisandra berries

By steadying the heart and easing emotional strain, Motherwort supports circulation guided by calm presence.

ROSE PETALS
rosa damascena

soften

HOW SHE MIGHT HELP
Emotional constriction, heart heaviness, and circulatory stagnation shaped by grief or stress often respond well to Rose, especially when softness and gentle movement support healing.

WORKING WITH HER
Gentle, consistent use allows Rose's soothing qualities to support emotional openness and circulatory ease. She is most often taken as an infusion or tincture and fits well into routines focused on heart-centered care. Ongoing relationship supports tenderness and balance.

AVOID COMBINING
Rose integrates smoothly with many heart-supportive herbs. Attentive pacing supports balance when layering with strongly astringent remedies used in high amounts.

IMPORTANT NOTES
Rose offers cooling, calming support and suits ongoing use. Beginning gently supports awareness of the body's response, particularly in emotional processing.

COMMON PREPARATIONS*

Tea (infusion)
Tincture
Syrup

*See the Preparation Guide in the back of this book

WORKS WELL WITH

hawthorn leaf and flower
hibiscus flower
motherwort
lemon balm
schisandra berries

Through softness and emotional nourishment, Rose supports the heart in opening and circulating with grace.

HIBISCUS FLOWER
hibiscus sabdariffa

cool

HOW SHE MIGHT HELP

Heat, circulatory tension, and cardiovascular strain often ease with Hibiscus, especially when cooling support and gentle movement benefit heart and vessel health.

WORKING WITH HER

Consistent, refreshing use allows Hibiscus's cooling and circulatory qualities to support flow and balance. She is most often taken as an infusion or syrup and fits well into routines focused on hydration and cardiovascular ease. Ongoing relationship supports lightness and clarity.

AVOID COMBINING

Hibiscus tends to feel most balanced when not layered heavily with other strongly cooling or diuretic remedies used in high amounts. Attentive pacing supports circulatory comfort.

IMPORTANT NOTES

Hibiscus offers cooling, gently astringent support and suits ongoing use. Beginning gently supports awareness of the body's response, particularly in blood pressure and hydration patterns.

COMMON PREPARATIONS*

Tea (infusion)
Syrup
Tincture

*See the Preparation Guide in the back of this book

WORKS WELL WITH

rose petals
hawthorn berry
lemon balm
schisandra berries
ginger

Through cooling movement and gentle nourishment, Hibiscus supports circulation shaped by balance and ease.

GINGER
zingiber officinale

circulate

HOW SHE MIGHT HELP
Coldness, stagnation, and sluggish circulation often respond to Ginger, especially when warmth and movement support cardiovascular flow.

WORKING WITH HER
Moderate, intentional use allows Ginger's warming qualities to encourage circulation and comfort. She is most often taken as an infusion, decoction, tincture, or food-based preparation and fits well into routines focused on restoring movement. Ongoing relationship supports vitality and warmth.

AVOID COMBINING
Ginger tends to feel most balanced when not layered heavily with other strongly heating remedies used in high amounts. Thoughtful attention supports comfort for those sensitive to heat.

IMPORTANT NOTES
Ginger carries an activating, warming nature and suits measured use. Beginning gently supports awareness of the body's response, particularly during periods of heat or inflammation.

COMMON PREPARATIONS*

Tea (infusion or decoction)
Tincture
Powder
Food-based preparations

*See the Preparation Guide in the back of this book

WORKS WELL WITH
turmeric
cayenne
hawthorn berry
garlic
schisandra berries

By encouraging warmth and movement, Ginger supports circulation that feels steady and alive.

TURMERIC
curcuma longa

circulate

HOW SHE MIGHT HELP
Inflammation affecting circulation and cardiovascular comfort often benefits from Turmeric, especially when steady anti-inflammatory support encourages ease of flow.

WORKING WITH HER
Consistent, mindful use allows Turmeric's balancing qualities to support vascular health over time. She is most often taken as a powder, tincture, or infusion and fits well into routines focused on long-term circulatory support. Ongoing relationship supports resilience and steadiness.

AVOID COMBINING
Turmeric tends to serve best when layered thoughtfully alongside other warming or blood-moving remedies. Attentive use also supports those working with anticoagulant medications.

IMPORTANT NOTES
Turmeric carries a warming, drying nature and suits measured use. Beginning gently supports clear observation of the body's response, particularly for those sensitive to heat.

COMMON PREPARATIONS*

Powder
Tincture
Tea (infusion or decoction)
Honey-based preparations

*See the Preparation Guide in the back of this book

WORKS WELL WITH

ginger
hawthorn berry
cayenne
garlic
schisandra berries

Through steady anti-inflammatory support, Turmeric helps circulation move with greater comfort and balance.

CAYENNE
capsicum annuum

circulate

HOW SHE MIGHT HELP

Poor circulation, cold extremities, and stagnation often respond to Cayenne, especially when rapid warming and movement support heart and vessel function.

WORKING WITH HER

Careful, minimal use allows Cayenne's stimulating qualities to activate circulation effectively. She is most often taken in very small internal doses or applied topically in salves and liniments. Thoughtful relationship supports benefit without excess intensity.

AVOID COMBINING

Cayenne tends to feel most balanced when not layered heavily with other strongly heating or stimulating remedies used in high amounts. Attentive pacing supports comfort and clarity.

IMPORTANT NOTES

Cayenne carries a strong activating nature and suits careful dosing. Beginning gently supports awareness of the body's response, particularly for sensitive systems.

COMMON PREPARATIONS*

Powder
Tincture
Salve or liniment

*See the Preparation Guide in the back of this book

WORKS WELL WITH

ginger
turmeric
hawthorn berry
garlic
schisandra berries

Through warmth and activation, Cayenne helps circulation reawaken and move with strength.

GARLIC
allium sativum

circulate

HOW SHE MIGHT HELP
Sluggish circulation, cardiovascular strain, and stagnation often respond well to Garlic, especially when warmth and movement support heart and vessel health.

WORKING WITH HER
Regular, moderate use allows Garlic's circulatory and protective qualities to support cardiovascular function. She is most often taken fresh, as a tincture, or incorporated into food and fits well into routines focused on daily heart support. Ongoing relationship supports resilience and flow.

AVOID COMBINING
Garlic tends to serve best when layered thoughtfully with other strong blood-moving remedies. Attentive use also supports those working with anticoagulant medications.

IMPORTANT NOTES
Garlic carries a warming, dispersing nature and suits consistent use. Beginning gently supports awareness of the body's response, particularly in digestion and circulation.

COMMON PREPARATIONS*

Fresh clove
Tincture
Food-based preparations

*See the Preparation Guide in the back of this book

WORKS WELL WITH

hawthorn berry
ginger
turmeric
cayenne
schisandra berries

Through warmth and steady movement, Garlic supports circulation that feels active and resilient.

GINKGO
ginkgo biloba

circulate

HOW SHE MIGHT HELP

Peripheral circulation challenges, mental fog, and reduced blood flow often ease with Ginkgo, especially when clarity and vascular support are needed together.

WORKING WITH HER

Consistent, attentive use allows Ginkgo's circulatory qualities to support blood flow to the brain and extremities. She is most often taken as a tincture or capsule and fits well into routines focused on cognitive clarity and vascular health. Ongoing relationship supports alert presence.

AVOID COMBINING

Ginkgo tends to feel most balanced when not layered heavily with other strong blood-thinning remedies. Thoughtful attention also serves those working with anticoagulant medications.

IMPORTANT NOTES

Ginkgo offers cooling, dispersing support and suits ongoing use. Beginning gently supports awareness of the body's response, particularly in circulation and focus.

COMMON PREPARATIONS*

Tincture
Capsule

*See the Preparation Guide in the back of this book

WORKS WELL WITH

schisandra berries
hawthorn leaf and flower
rosemary
ginger
yarrow

By supporting clear blood flow, Ginkgo helps circulation reach where it is most needed.

YARROW
achillea millefolium

regulate — III

HOW SHE MIGHT HELP
Circulatory stagnation, temperature imbalance, and uneven flow often respond well to Yarrow, especially when gentle regulation supports balance.

WORKING WITH HER
Moderate, consistent use allows Yarrow's regulating qualities to support circulation without excess stimulation. She is most often taken as an infusion or tincture and fits well into routines focused on restoring balance and flow. Ongoing relationship supports steadiness.

AVOID COMBINING
Yarrow tends to feel most balanced when not layered heavily with other strong blood-moving or drying remedies used in high amounts. Attentive pacing supports comfort.

IMPORTANT NOTES
Yarrow carries a drying, harmonizing nature and suits measured use. Beginning gently supports awareness of the body's response, particularly during shifts in circulation.

COMMON PREPARATIONS*

Tea (infusion)
Tincture

*See the Preparation Guide in the back of this book

WORKS WELL WITH

hawthorn leaf and flower
ginger
ginkgo
rose petals
motherwort

Through regulation and balance, Yarrow helps circulation settle into a steady rhythm.

SCHISANDRA BERRIES
schisandra chinensis

tone

HOW SHE MIGHT HELP

Circulatory fatigue, stress-related strain, and difficulty sustaining vascular tone often respond well to Schisandra, especially when endurance and adaptability support heart health.

WORKING WITH HER

Consistent, intentional use allows Schisandra's adaptogenic qualities to support circulation and cardiovascular resilience. She is most often taken as a tincture, decoction, or powder and fits well into routines focused on steady strength. Ongoing relationship supports durability and focus.

AVOID COMBINING

Schisandra tends to feel most balanced when not layered heavily with multiple stimulating adaptogens used at the same time. Thoughtful pacing supports clarity.

IMPORTANT NOTES

Schisandra carries a tonifying, strengthening nature and suits ongoing use. Beginning gently supports awareness of the body's response, particularly in sleep and circulation.

COMMON PREPARATIONS*

Tea (decoction)
Tincture
Powder

*See the Preparation Guide in the back of this book

WORKS WELL WITH

hawthorn berry
ginkgo
eleuthero
rosemary
garlic

By supporting endurance and vascular tone, Schisandra helps circulation remain strong under sustained demand.

RED SAGE ROOT (DANSHEN)

salvia miltiorrhiza

HOW SHE MIGHT HELP

Deep circulatory stagnation, cardiovascular tension, and patterns shaped by long-term strain often respond well to Red Sage Root, especially when movement and nourishment need to occur together.

WORKING WITH HER

Measured, consistent use allows Red Sage Root's blood-moving and restorative qualities to support circulation at a deeper level. She is most often taken as a decoction, tincture, or capsule and fits well into routines focused on long-view cardiovascular balance. Ongoing relationship supports renewal and flow.

AVOID COMBINING

Red Sage Root tends to serve best when not layered heavily with other strong blood-moving or anticoagulant remedies. Thoughtful attention also supports those working with cardiovascular medications.

IMPORTANT NOTES

Red Sage Root carries a cooling, dispersing nature and suits steady, intentional use. Beginning gently supports awareness of the body's response, particularly in circulation and recovery patterns.

---

renew

COMMON PREPARATIONS*

Tea (decoction)
Tincture
Capsule

*See the Preparation Guide in the back of this book

WORKS WELL WITH

hawthorn berry
schisandra berries
turmeric
ginkgo
rose petals

By encouraging movement and renewal at depth, Red Sage Root supports circulation shaped by restoration and balance.

ROSEMARY
salvia rosmarinus

circulate

HOW SHE MIGHT HELP

Sluggish circulation, mental heaviness, and diminished warmth often lift with Rosemary, especially when clarity and movement support heart and vessel vitality.

WORKING WITH HER

Intentional, moderate use allows Rosemary's aromatic and circulatory qualities to support alertness and flow. She is most often taken as an infusion, tincture, or aromatic preparation and fits well into routines focused on stimulation with purpose. Thoughtful relationship supports clarity and warmth.

AVOID COMBINING

Rosemary tends to feel most balanced when not layered heavily with other strongly stimulating remedies used in high amounts. Attentive pacing supports comfort for those sensitive to activation.

IMPORTANT NOTES

Rosemary carries a warming, activating nature and suits measured use. Beginning gently supports awareness of the body's response, particularly in circulation and nervous system tone.

COMMON PREPARATIONS*

Tea (infusion)
Tincture
Steam or aromatic use

*See the Preparation Guide in the back of this book

WORKS WELL WITH

ginkgo
ginger
schisandra berries
hawthorn leaf and flower
garlic

Through warmth, clarity, and movement, Rosemary helps circulation feel awake, supported, and alive.

SECTION EIGHT

SKIN & LYMPH DETOX

The skin and lymphatic system reflect how the body clears waste, responds to congestion, and maintains internal balance. Lymph moves slowly and steadily, relying on hydration, movement, breath, and healthy circulation to support detoxification and immune awareness. When these systems feel supported, the skin often becomes clearer, tissues feel lighter, and overall vitality improves.

The remedies gathered here support detoxification through gentle, sustained pathways. Some encourage lymphatic movement, helping clear stagnation and reduce swelling or congestion beneath the surface. Others nourish and protect the skin, soothing irritation while supporting repair and renewal. Several work through the liver, kidneys, and blood, illustrating how detoxification unfolds as a coordinated process rather than a single action. Together, these plants reflect the close relationship between internal cleansing and outward expression through the skin.

Leaves, roots, flowers, and warming spices appear throughout these pages because of their long-standing use in supporting elimination and tissue health across cultures and traditions. They demonstrate foundational detox patterns such as moving and draining, cooling and soothing, warming and activating. Working with them reveals how detoxification responds to consistency, patience, and gentle encouragement rather than force.

These pages invite attentiveness to texture, tone, swelling, and flow. Observing changes in skin, lymph, and overall lightness becomes a form of listening, guided by plants that have long supported the body's natural clearing processes. May this collection offer a steady entry point into skin and lymph support and deepen understanding of the rhythms that allow cleansing and renewal to occur with ease.

cleavers
calendula
red clover
burdock root
dandelion root
dandelion leaf
nettle leaf
violet leaf
chickweed
yellow dock
poke root
ginger
cayenne
echinacea

CLEAVERS
galium aparine

movement

HOW SHE MIGHT HELP

Lymphatic congestion, swelling, and skin issues linked to stagnation often ease with Cleavers, especially when gentle movement and drainage support relief.

WORKING WITH HER

Light, consistent use allows Cleavers' cooling and moving qualities to encourage lymphatic flow. She is most often taken as a fresh infusion or tincture and fits well into routines focused on softening congestion. Ongoing relationship supports lightness and ease.

AVOID COMBINING

Cleavers generally integrates smoothly with many detox-supportive herbs. Attentive pacing supports balance when layering with strong diuretics used in high amounts.

IMPORTANT NOTES

Cleavers carries a cooling, moistening nature and suits gentle, ongoing use. Beginning slowly supports clear awareness of the body's response, particularly for those sensitive to cooling effects.

COMMON PREPARATIONS*

Tea (infusion)
Tincture
Fresh juice

*See the Preparation Guide in the back of this book

WORKS WELL WITH

calendula
violet leaf
burdock root
nettle leaf
red clover

By encouraging lymphatic movement, Cleavers supports the body in releasing congestion and restoring flow.

CALENDULA
calendula officinalis

soothe

HOW SHE MIGHT HELP

Skin irritation, sluggish lymph, and inflammation beneath the surface often respond well to Calendula, especially when gentle repair and cleansing support are needed together.

WORKING WITH HER

Steady, soothing use allows Calendula's restorative qualities to support lymphatic and skin health. She is most often taken as an infusion, tincture, or topical preparation and fits well into routines focused on calming and renewal. Ongoing relationship supports resilience.

AVOID COMBINING

Calendula integrates smoothly with many skin- and lymph-supportive herbs. Attentive use supports balance when layering with strongly stimulating remedies used topically.

IMPORTANT NOTES

Calendula offers gentle, nourishing support and suits ongoing use. Beginning gently supports awareness of the body's response, particularly for sensitive or reactive skin.

COMMON PREPARATIONS*

Tea (infusion)
Tincture
Salve or infused oil

*See the Preparation Guide in the back of this book

WORKS WELL WITH

cleavers
violet leaf
chickweed
burdock root
dandelion leaf

Through soothing and renewal, Calendula supports healthy skin and lymphatic balance.

RED CLOVER
trifolium pratense

cleanse   118

HOW SHE MIGHT HELP
Chronic skin issues, lymphatic stagnation, and systemic congestion often benefit from Red Clover, especially when gentle cleansing supports long-term balance.

WORKING WITH HER
Consistent, long-view use allows Red Clover's cleansing qualities to support lymphatic and blood health. She is most often taken as an infusion or tincture and fits well into routines focused on gradual detoxification. Ongoing relationship supports clarity and ease.

AVOID COMBINING
Red Clover generally integrates smoothly with many detox-supportive herbs. Thoughtful pacing supports balance when layering with concentrated phytoestrogenic remedies used in high amounts.

IMPORTANT NOTES
Red Clover carries a cooling, cleansing nature and suits steady use. Beginning gently supports observation of the body's response over time.

COMMON PREPARATIONS*

Tea (infusion)
Tincture

*See the Preparation Guide in the back of this book

WORKS WELL WITH
burdock root
cleavers
nettle leaf
yellow dock
violet leaf

By supporting gentle cleansing and circulation, Red Clover helps the body clear congestion reflected through the skin.

BURDOCK ROOT
arctium lappa

nourish

HOW SHE MIGHT HELP

Persistent skin conditions, inflammatory congestion, and sluggish elimination often respond well to Burdock, especially when deep cleansing and nourishment support detoxification.

WORKING WITH HER

Steady, patient use allows Burdock's grounding qualities to support lymph, blood, and liver pathways together. She is most often taken as a decoction, tincture, or food-based preparation and fits well into routines focused on sustained detox support. Ongoing relationship supports resilience.

AVOID COMBINING

Burdock integrates smoothly with many detox-supportive herbs. Attentive use supports balance when layering with strong diuretics used in high amounts.

IMPORTANT NOTES

Burdock suits consistent, moderate use and is typically well tolerated. Beginning gently supports awareness of the body's response during periods of cleansing.

COMMON PREPARATIONS*

Tea (decoction)
Tincture
Food-based preparations

*See the Preparation Guide in the back of this book

WORKS WELL WITH

red clover
yellow dock
dandelion root
cleavers
nettle leaf

Through deep nourishment and cleansing support, Burdock helps the body clear congestion and restore skin vitality.

DANDELION ROOT
taraxacum officinale

eliminate

HOW SHE MIGHT HELP

Deep-seated congestion, sluggish elimination, and skin issues linked to liver and lymph stagnation often respond well to Dandelion Root, especially when steady cleansing supports balance.

WORKING WITH HER

Consistent, long-view use allows Dandelion Root's grounding qualities to support liver and lymph pathways together. She is most often taken as a decoction, tincture, or food-based preparation and fits well into routines focused on sustained detoxification. Ongoing relationship supports resilience and clarity.

AVOID COMBINING

Dandelion Root generally integrates smoothly with many detox-supportive herbs. Attentive pacing supports balance when layering with strong bitter tonics used in high amounts.

IMPORTANT NOTES

Dandelion Root carries a warming, grounding nature and suits ongoing use. Beginning gently supports awareness of the body's response, particularly during periods of cleansing.

COMMON PREPARATIONS*

Tea (decoction)
Tincture
Food-based preparations

*See the Preparation Guide in the back of this book

WORKS WELL WITH

burdock root
yellow dock
red clover
cleavers
nettle leaf

By supporting deep elimination pathways, Dandelion Root helps the body clear congestion reflected through the skin.

DANDELION LEAF
taraxacum officinale

HOW SHE MIGHT HELP

Fluid retention, lymphatic swelling, and skin puffiness often ease with Dandelion Leaf, especially when gentle drainage supports detoxification.

WORKING WITH HER

Light, consistent use allows Dandelion Leaf's moving qualities to support lymphatic flow and kidney function. She is most often taken as an infusion or tincture and fits well into routines focused on releasing excess fluid. Ongoing relationship supports lightness and ease.

AVOID COMBINING

Dandelion Leaf tends to feel most balanced when not layered heavily with other strong diuretics used in high amounts. Attentive pacing supports hydration balance.

IMPORTANT NOTES

Dandelion Leaf carries a cooling, draining nature and suits gentle use. Beginning slowly supports clear observation of the body's response, particularly in electrolyte balance.

---

detox

COMMON PREPARATIONS*

Tea (infusion)
Tincture
Fresh leaf preparations

*See the Preparation Guide in the back of this book

WORKS WELL WITH

cleavers
violet leaf
nettle leaf
calendula
red clover

Through gentle drainage and movement, Dandelion Leaf supports lymphatic clarity and skin vitality.

NETTLE LEAF
urtica dioica

nourish

HOW SHE MIGHT HELP
Inflammatory skin conditions, nutrient depletion, and sluggish lymph often benefit from Nettle Leaf, especially when nourishment and cleansing support are needed together.

WORKING WITH HER
Steady, nourishing use allows Nettle Leaf's mineral-rich qualities to support detox pathways without depletion. She is most often taken as an infusion or food-based preparation and fits well into routines focused on rebuilding and cleansing simultaneously. Ongoing relationship supports strength and balance.

AVOID COMBINING
Nettle Leaf generally integrates smoothly with many detox-supportive herbs. Thoughtful pacing supports balance when layering with strong diuretics used in high amounts.

IMPORTANT NOTES
Nettle Leaf suits ongoing use and is typically well tolerated. Beginning gently supports awareness of the body's response, particularly during periods of increased elimination.

COMMON PREPARATIONS*

Tea (infusion)
Food-based preparations
Tincture

*See the Preparation Guide in the back of this book

WORKS WELL WITH
red clover
burdock root
dandelion leaf
violet leaf
yellow dock

By nourishing while cleansing, Nettle Leaf supports skin and lymph health with steadiness and strength.

VIOLET LEAF
viola odorata

soothe

HOW SHE MIGHT HELP
Heat, irritation, and congested lymph reflected through the skin often soften with Violet Leaf, especially when cooling and soothing support ease.

WORKING WITH HER
Gentle, patient use allows Violet Leaf's cooling qualities to support lymphatic movement and skin comfort. She is most often taken as an infusion, syrup, or topical preparation and fits well into routines focused on calming and softening. Ongoing relationship supports relief and balance.

AVOID COMBINING
Violet Leaf tends to feel most balanced when not layered heavily with other strongly cooling remedies used in high amounts. Attentive pacing supports comfort.

IMPORTANT NOTES
Violet Leaf carries a cooling, moistening nature and suits gentle, ongoing use. Beginning slowly supports awareness of the body's response, particularly for sensitive skin.

COMMON PREPARATIONS*

Tea (infusion)
Syrup
Salve or infused oil

*See the Preparation Guide in the back of this book

WORKS WELL WITH

cleavers
calendula
dandelion leaf
nettle leaf
chickweed

Through cooling and gentle movement, Violet Leaf supports skin and lymph in returning to ease.

CHICKWEED
stellaria media

move

HOW SHE MIGHT HELP

Heat, irritation, and congested skin conditions often soften with Chickweed, especially when cooling and soothing support lymphatic flow.

WORKING WITH HER

Gentle, consistent use allows Chickweed's calming qualities to support skin comfort and lymphatic ease. She is most often taken as an infusion, fresh preparation, or topical application and fits well into routines focused on softening irritation. Ongoing relationship supports relief and balance.

AVOID COMBINING

Chickweed tends to feel most balanced when not layered heavily with other strongly cooling remedies used in high amounts. Attentive pacing supports comfort.

IMPORTANT NOTES

Chickweed carries a cooling, moistening nature and suits gentle, ongoing use. Beginning slowly supports clear observation of the body's response, particularly for sensitive skin.

COMMON PREPARATIONS*

Tea (infusion)
Fresh plant preparations
Salve or poultice

*See the Preparation Guide in the back of this book

WORKS WELL WITH

violet leaf
calendula
cleavers
nettle leaf
red clover

Through cooling relief and gentle movement, Chickweed supports skin and lymph in settling and clearing.

YELLOW DOCK
rumex crispus

eliminate

HOW SHE MIGHT HELP

Chronic skin concerns, sluggish elimination, and lymphatic congestion often benefit from Yellow Dock, especially when gentle stimulation supports detox pathways.

WORKING WITH HER

Steady, moderate use allows Yellow Dock's bitter and cleansing qualities to support liver and lymph function together. She is most often taken as a decoction or tincture and fits well into routines focused on gradual detoxification. Ongoing relationship supports clarity and flow.

AVOID COMBINING

Yellow Dock tends to serve best when not layered heavily with other strong laxative or bitter remedies used in high amounts. Thoughtful pacing supports digestive comfort.

IMPORTANT NOTES

Yellow Dock carries a stimulating, grounding nature and suits measured use. Beginning gently supports awareness of the body's response, particularly in digestion and elimination.

COMMON PREPARATIONS*

Tea (decoction)
Tincture

*See the Preparation Guide in the back of this book

WORKS WELL WITH

burdock root
red clover
dandelion root
nettle leaf
cleavers

By supporting elimination and movement, Yellow Dock helps clear congestion reflected through the skin.

POKE ROOT
(LOW-DOSE, PRACTITIONER-GUIDED)

phytolacca americana

move

HOW SHE MIGHT HELP

Deep lymphatic congestion, swelling, and hardened tissue patterns may respond to Poke Root, especially when gentle yet focused movement is required.

WORKING WITH HER

Careful, practitioner-guided use allows Poke Root's powerful lymph-moving qualities to support deep clearing. She is most often taken as a very low-dose tincture and fits well into short, intentional protocols rather than ongoing routines. Respectful relationship supports effectiveness with safety.

AVOID COMBINING

Poke Root serves best when not layered with other strong lymphatic stimulants or aggressive detox remedies. Thoughtful guidance supports clarity and balance.

IMPORTANT NOTES

Poke Root is a potent plant and requires skilled oversight. Use remains limited to very small amounts for short durations, with close attention to the body's response.

COMMON PREPARATIONS*

Low-dose tincture only

*See the Preparation Guide in the back of this book

WORKS WELL WITH

cleavers
red clover
echinacea (lymphatic use)
burdock root

Through deep, directed movement, Poke Root supports lymphatic clearing when guided with care and respect.

GINGER
zingiber officinale

flow

HOW SHE MIGHT HELP
Sluggish lymphatic movement and cold-related congestion often respond well to Ginger, especially when warmth supports circulation and flow.

WORKING WITH HER
Moderate, consistent use allows Ginger's warming qualities to stimulate lymphatic and circulatory movement. She is most often taken as an infusion, decoction, tincture, or food-based preparation and fits well into routines focused on activation with balance. Ongoing relationship supports momentum and ease.

AVOID COMBINING
Ginger tends to feel most balanced when not layered heavily with other strongly heating remedies used in high amounts. Attentive pacing supports comfort for sensitive systems.

IMPORTANT NOTES
Ginger carries an activating, warming nature and suits measured use. Beginning gently supports awareness of the body's response, particularly during inflammatory or heated states.

COMMON PREPARATIONS*

Tea (infusion or decoction)
Tincture
Powder
Food-based preparations

*See the Preparation Guide in the back of this book

WORKS WELL WITH

burdock root
yellow dock
cayenne
echinacea (lymphatic use)
schisandra berries

Through warmth and movement, Ginger helps lymph and circulation regain steady flow.

CAYENNE
capsicum annuum

flow

HOW SHE MIGHT HELP

Sluggish lymphatic flow, cold stagnation, and congested tissues often respond to Cayenne, especially when warmth and circulation support movement and clearing.

WORKING WITH HER

Careful, minimal use allows Cayenne's stimulating qualities to activate lymphatic and circulatory pathways. She is most often taken in very small internal amounts or applied topically in salves and liniments. Thoughtful relationship supports effectiveness without overwhelm.

AVOID COMBINING

Cayenne tends to serve best when not layered heavily with other strongly heating or stimulating remedies used in high amounts. Attentive pacing supports comfort and balance.

IMPORTANT NOTES

Cayenne carries a strong activating nature and suits careful dosing. Beginning gently supports awareness of the body's response, particularly for sensitive systems or inflamed states.

COMMON PREPARATIONS*

Powder
Tincture
Salve or liniment

*See the Preparation Guide in the back of this book

WORKS WELL WITH

ginger
burdock root
echinacea (lymphatic use)
garlic
schisandra berries

Through warmth and activation, Cayenne helps lymphatic flow reawaken and move with strength.

ECHINACEA
(LYMPHATIC USE)

echinacea angustifolia

HOW SHE MIGHT HELP

Swollen lymph nodes, stagnation, and immune congestion often respond well to Echinacea when used with a lymphatic focus, especially during periods of acute challenge.

WORKING WITH HER

Short-term, attentive use allows Echinacea's stimulating and immune-supportive qualities to engage lymphatic movement. She is most often taken as a tincture and fits well into focused protocols rather than long-term routines. Thoughtful relationship supports responsiveness and clarity.

AVOID COMBINING

Echinacea tends to serve best when not layered heavily with other strong immune stimulants used at the same time. Attentive pacing supports balance during active protocols.

IMPORTANT NOTES

Echinacea carries a stimulating, mobilizing nature and suits targeted use. Beginning gently supports awareness of the body's response, particularly in immune and lymphatic systems.

---

flow

COMMON PREPARATIONS*

Tincture

*See the Preparation Guide in the back of this book

WORKS WELL WITH

cleavers
poke root (low-dose, practitioner-guided)
calendula
ginger
red clover

By mobilizing lymph and immune response, Echinacea supports the body during moments that call for clear, active defense.

PREPARATION GUIDE

Working With Plant Preparations

The way a plant is prepared shapes how it meets the body. An infusion carries a different conversation than a tincture. A poultice offers direct engagement with tissue. A powder moves gently through daily rhythms. Each preparation provides its own pathway of relationship, expression, and support.

This guide offers orientation and context for the preparations referenced throughout this book. The methods shared here reflect time-tested ways of working with plants and support thoughtful choice based on body awareness, capacity, and the moment at hand.

Working with one or two familiar preparations creates a strong foundation for meaningful relationship with plant medicine and allows understanding to grow naturally over time.

The preparation methods described offer many doorways into relationship with plants. Trust grows through listening, consistency, and attention. The plants meet each person differently, and the most supportive approach is often the one that fits naturally into daily life.

infusions (tea)

decoctions

tinctures

powders

capsules

syrups

honey- & ghee-based preparations

food-based preparations

topical preparations
(salve, oil, poultice, compress)

steam or aromatic uses

low-dose/practitioner-guided preparations

PREPARATION GUIDE

INFUSIONS (Tea)

What it is:
An infusion is made by steeping plant material in hot water (not boiling), allowing the soluble properties of the plant to gently release.

When it's often chosen:
Infusions are commonly used for daily support, nourishment, and gradual regulation. They suit leaves, flowers, and gentle herbs that offer their medicine readily.

What to know:
Infusions invite consistency and presence. Fresh or dried plant material may be used, depending on availability and preference.

Typical timing:
Often worked with throughout the day or in the evening, depending on the plant.

EXAMPLE PREPARATION

Place one tablespoon dried herb or a small handful of fresh herb in a jar or mug. Pour hot (not boiling) water over the plant, cover, and steep for 10–20 minutes. Strain and drink.

infusions (tea)

decoctions

tinctures

powders

capsules

syrups

honey- & ghee-based preparations

food-based preparations

topical preparations
(salve, oil, poultice, compress)

steam or aromatic uses

low-dose/practitioner-guided preparations

PREPARATION GUIDE

DECOCTIONS

What it is:
A decoction involves simmering tougher plant material such as roots, bark, or berries to draw out deeper constituents.

When it's often chosen:
Decoctions are frequently selected for grounding, strengthening, or long-term support, especially with roots and dense plant parts.

What to know:
This method carries a slower, more concentrated feel and pairs well with plants that benefit from heat and time.

Typical timing:
Often taken earlier in the day or used in focused periods rather than continuously.

EXAMPLE PREPARATION

Add one tablespoon dried root, bark, or berry to a small pot with 2 cups of water. Bring to a gentle simmer, cover, and cook for 20–30 minutes. Strain before drinking.

infusions (tea)

decoctions

tinctures

powders

capsules

syrups

honey- & ghee-based preparations

food-based preparations

topical preparations
(salve, oil, poultice, compress)

steam or aromatic uses

low-dose/practitioner-guided preparations

PREPARATION GUIDE

TINCTURES

What are they:
Tinctures are either alcohol- or glycerin-based extractions that concentrate plant properties into liquid form.

When they're often chosen:
Tinctures are commonly used when flexibility, portability, or precise dosing is helpful.

What to know:
A small amount carries a strong presence. Tinctures allow for short-term use or ongoing support, depending on the plant.

Typical timing:
Used as needed or taken consistently, guided by the plant's nature.

EXAMPLE PREPARATION

Fill a glass jar halfway with chopped dried or fresh plant material. Cover completely with alcohol (80-100 proof, clear - <u>not</u> rubbing alcohol) or glycerin, seal, and store in a dark place for several weeks, shaking occasionally. Strain and bottle.

---

infusions (tea)

decoctions

tinctures

powders

capsules

syrups

honey- & ghee-based preparations

food-based preparations

topical preparations
(salve, oil, poultice, compress)

steam or aromatic uses

low-dose/practitioner-guided preparations

PREPARATION GUIDE

POWDERS

What are they:
Powders are finely ground plant material taken directly or blended into food or drink.

When they're often chosen:
Powders are often used for nutritive herbs and tonics that support long-term vitality.

What to know:
This method works slowly and steadily, integrating easily into daily routines.

Typical timing:
Often taken in the morning or alongside meals.

EXAMPLE PREPARATION

Use finely ground plant powder as is or mix into warm water, tea, honey, or food. A small amount taken consistently supports gradual integration.

infusions (tea)

decoctions

tinctures

powders

capsules

syrups

honey- & ghee-based preparations

food-based preparations

topical preparations
(salve, oil, poultice, compress)

steam or aromatic uses

low-dose/practitioner-guided preparations

PREPARATION GUIDE

CAPSULES

What are they:
Capsules contain powdered plant material in a measured form.

When they're often chosen:
Capsules offer convenience and neutrality of taste.

What to know:
This preparation favors consistency and ease over sensory engagement.

Typical timing:
Typically taken with meals or at regular intervals.

EXAMPLE PREPARATION

Place powdered plant material into empty capsules using a capsule-filling tray or by hand. Store in a labeled container and take as part of a regular routine.

infusions (tea)

decoctions

tinctures

powders

capsules

syrups

honey- & ghee-based preparations

food-based preparations

topical preparations
(salve, oil, poultice, compress)

steam or aromatic uses

low-dose/practitioner-guided preparations

PREPARATION GUIDE

SYRUPS

What are they:
Syrups combine plant infusions or decoctions with a sweet base, often honey.

When they're often chosen:
Syrups are commonly used for respiratory, immune, or throat support.

What to know:
This method carries a soothing, accessible quality and is often well received across ages.

Typical timing:
Used as needed or during focused periods of support.

EXAMPLE PREPARATION

Prepare a strong infusion or decoction, then gently warm with honey until blended. Store in a glass jar in the refrigerator and use as needed.

infusions (tea)

decoctions

tinctures

powders

capsules

syrups

honey- & ghee-based preparations

food-based preparations

topical preparations
(salve, oil, poultice, compress)

steam or aromatic uses

low-dose/practitioner-guided preparations

PREPARATION GUIDE

HONEY- & GHEE-BASED PREPARATIONS

What are they:
Plant material is infused into honey or ghee in order to create a nourishing, preserved preparation.

When they're often chosen:
These forms suit tonic herbs and plants that benefit from slow assimilation.

What to know:
They pair well with rituals of nourishment and daily care.

Typical timing:
Often taken in small amounts, regularly.

infusions (tea)

decoctions

tinctures

powders

capsules

syrups

honey- & ghee-based preparations

food-based preparations

topical preparations
(salve, oil, poultice, compress)

steam or aromatic uses

low-dose/practitioner-guided preparations

EXAMPLE PREPARATIONS

Honey: Cover dried herbs completely with honey in a glass jar. Stir to release air bubbles, seal, and allow to infuse for several weeks. Use by the spoonful as desired.

Ghee: Warm ghee gently and add finely chopped dried herb. Keep on low heat for several hours, then strain and store. Use in small amounts as part of daily nourishment.

PREPARATION GUIDE

FOOD-BASED PREPARATIONS

What are they:
Plants are incorporated directly into meals, broths, or culinary preparations.

When they're often chosen:
This approach supports gentle, long-term integration of plant medicine into daily life.

What to know:
Used regularly, as part of meals.

Typical timing:
Often taken in small amounts, regularly.

EXAMPLE PREPARATION

Add herbs directly to soups, broths, grains, or other meals during cooking. Consistent inclusion supports gentle, long-term relationship with the plant.

infusions (tea)

decoctions

tinctures

powders

capsules

syrups

honey- & ghee-based preparations

food-based preparations

topical preparations
(salve, oil, poultice, compress)

steam or aromatic uses

low-dose/practitioner-guided preparations

PREPARATION GUIDE

TOPICAL PREPARATIONS

What are they:
Salves, oils, poultices, and compresses applied directly to the body.

When they're often chosen:
Topicals are used for localized support involving skin, muscles, joints, or lymph.

What to know:
This method offers direct engagement with tissue and sensation.

Typical timing:
Applied as needed or in short-term support cycles.

EXAMPLE PREPARATION

Infuse herbs in oil over low heat or time, then strain and apply directly to skin. Fresh herbs may also be crushed and applied as a poultice for localized support.

infusions (tea)

decoctions

tinctures

powders

capsules

syrups

honey- & ghee-based preparations

food-based preparations

topical preparations
(salve, oil, poultice, compress)

steam or aromatic uses

low-dose/practitioner-guided preparations

PREPARATION GUIDE

STEAM or AROMATIC USES

What are they:
Plant vapors or aromas inhaled through steam or ambient diffusion.

When they're often chosen:
This method supports respiratory, emotional, and circulatory pathways.

What to know:
Aromatic preparations work quickly and subtly through breath and nervous system response.

Typical timing:
Often used in the moment or during intentional rest.

EXAMPLE PREPARATION

Place aromatic herbs in a bowl and pour hot water over them. Lean over the bowl, cover head loosely with a towel, and breathe the steam for several minutes.

---

infusions (tea)

decoctions

tinctures

powders

capsules

syrups

honey- & ghee-based preparations

food-based preparations

topical preparations
(salve, oil, poultice, compress)

steam or aromatic uses

low-dose/practitioner-guided preparations

PREPARATION GUIDE

LOW-DOSE, PRACTITIONER GUIDED

What are they:
Certain plants carry strong actions and are traditionally worked with in very small amounts under skilled guidance.

When they're often chosen:
These preparations appear in the book only when appropriate and are clearly marked.

What to know:
Respect and discernment guide these relationships.

Typical timing:
Short-term, intentional use.

EXAMPLE PREPARATION

Prepare only under the guidance of a trained practitioner using very small, measured amounts. These preparations are used intentionally and for short periods.

infusions (tea)

decoctions

tinctures

powders

capsules

syrups

honey-based preparations

ghee-based preparations

food-based preparations

topical preparations
(salve, oil, poultice, compress)

steam or aromatic uses

low-dose/practitioner-guided preparations

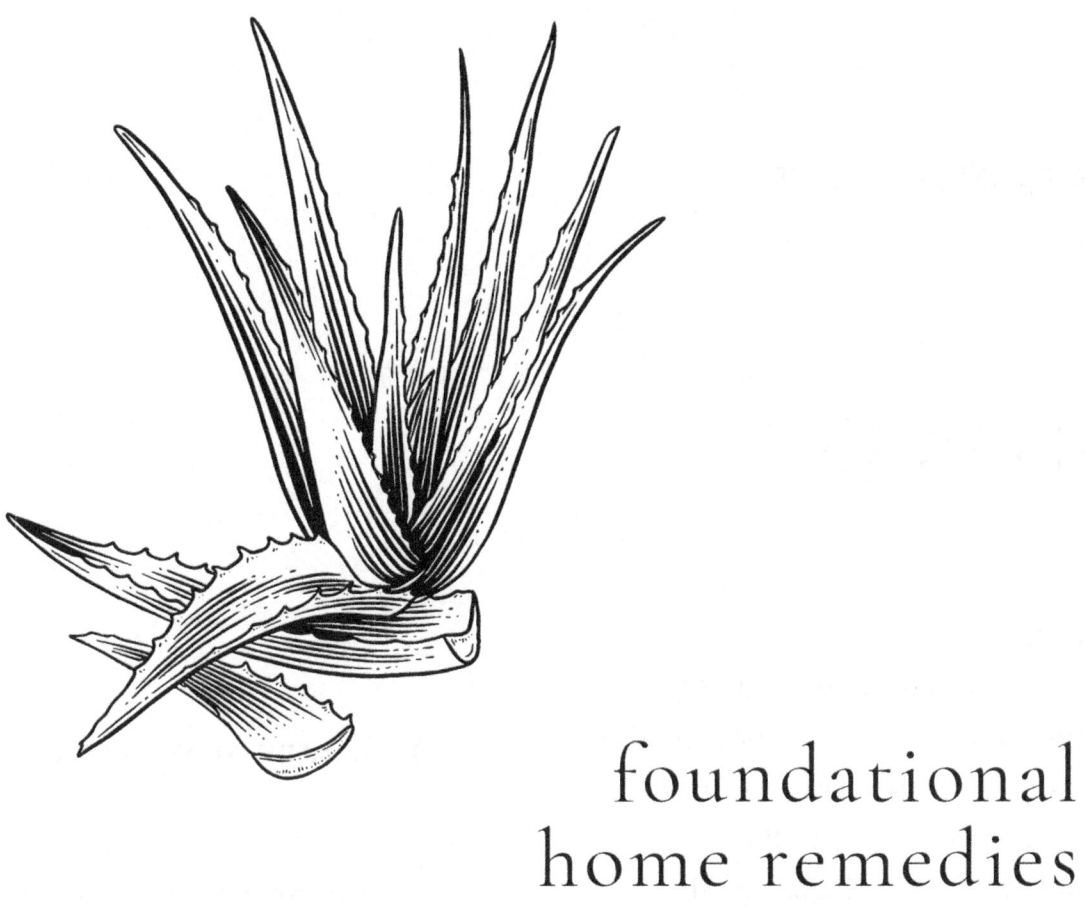

foundational home remedies

The remedies gathered here offer simple, effective ways to support the body using materials that are often already within reach. They work through warmth, cooling, drawing, nourishment, and gentle stimulation. These approaches have supported households and communities for generations through attentiveness, consistency, and respect for the body's signals.

This section offers orientation and practical starting points rather than fixed protocols. Each remedy invites observation, patience, and responsiveness. Used with care, these practices support comfort, circulation, and recovery while strengthening trust in the body's capacity to respond.

FOUNDATIONAL HOME REMEDIES

CASTOR OIL

Why it's used:
Castor oil has long been worked with to encourage circulation, soften stagnation, and support tissue comfort. Applied externally, it offers steady warmth and depth that supports lymphatic flow and local relief.

Basic preparation:
A clean cloth is saturated with castor oil and placed over the area receiving support. Gentle warmth may be added, and the body is allowed to rest during application.

Use rhythm:
Used several times per week or in short series, guided by comfort and response.

Notes:
External use supports ease and effectiveness through steady, attentive practice.

primary support areas

pain and inflammation
lymphatic movement
pelvic and abdominal support
hemorrhoid comfort

FOUNDATIONAL HOME REMEDIES

POTATO POULTICE

Why they're used:
Potatoes have been traditionally worked with to draw out heat and soothe inflamed tissue. Their cooling, drawing action supports comfort during periods of acute irritation.

Basic preparation:
Raw potato is grated or sliced and placed on clean cloth, then applied directly to the area receiving support. Wrap the entire area and allow it to rest. Refresh poultice as needed.

Use rhythm:
Used as needed during periods of active discomfort. Best if you can leave in place for at least two hours; overnight is ideal.

Notes:
Fresh preparation supports clarity and responsiveness

primary support areas

pain and inflammation
heat and swelling
bruising and tissue irritation
hemorrhoid comfort

FOUNDATIONAL HOME REMEDIES

ALOE VERA

Why it's used:
Aloe vera has a long history of supporting cooling, soothing, and hydration. Its gel supports comfort both externally and internally when prepared appropriately.

Basic preparation:
Fresh aloe gel is applied directly to the skin or carefully prepared for internal use using food-grade aloe.

Use rhythm:
Used as needed or in short series, guided by sensation and response.

Notes:
Clear distinction between external and internal use supports safe, effective practice.

primary support areas

skin irritation and burns
digestive soothing
tissue hydration
hemorrhoid comfort

FOUNDATIONAL HOME REMEDIES

WOMB ELECTUARY
HONEY PASTE

Why it's used:
Electuaries combine herbs with honey to create nourishing, slowly absorbed support. Womb-focused blends have traditionally supported cycles of change through nourishment and warmth.

Basic preparation:
Finely powdered herbs are blended with honey to form a smooth paste and stored in a sealed jar.

Use rhythm:
Taken in small amounts regularly during supportive phases.

Notes:
Consistency and simplicity support the deepest benefit.

primary support areas

hormonal and cyclical comfort
pelvic nourishment
fatigue and depletion
emotional steadiness

FOUNDATIONAL HOME REMEDIES

SALT WATER / SALINE

Why it's used:
Salt water supports cleansing and comfort through mineral balance. Its use spans cultures and traditions as a foundational care practice.

Basic preparation:
Salt is dissolved in clean water to create a mild saline solution appropriate to the area being supported.

Use rhythm:
Used as needed with gentle attention.

Notes:
Clean water and appropriate ratios support comfort and clarity.

primary support areas

wound cleansing
throat comfort
nasal and sinus support
eye and skin rinses

FOUNDATIONAL HOME REMEDIES

WARM COMPRESS

Why it's used:
Warmth encourages circulation, relaxation, and containment. Compresses offer direct, comforting support to areas requesting ease.

Basic preparation:
A cloth is warmed in water, wrung out, and placed over the body with attention to comfort.

Use rhythm:
Used during rest or when tension or heaviness is present.

Notes:
Gentle warmth supports relaxation and responsiveness.

primary support areas

muscle tension
cramping
lymphatic stagnation
abdominal and pelvic comfort

FOUNDATIONAL HOME REMEDIES

COLD COMPRESS

Why it's used:
Cooling supports constriction and settling during periods of heat or swelling. Cold compresses offer timely relief when tissues feel overstimulated.

Basic preparation:
A cool, damp cloth is applied to the area receiving support.

Use rhythm:
Used in short applications during periods of heat or swelling.

Notes:
Attentive timing supports comfort and balance.

primary support areas

acute inflammation
swelling
headache support
recent injury

Alternating warm and cool compresses:

- This practice uses a longer period of warmth followed by a brief period of cooling. **Warmth** is applied for approximately **three minutes** to encourage circulation and relaxation.
- **Cooling follows for approximately thirty seconds** to support toning and responsiveness.

The cycle may be **repeated three times** (as needed), guided by comfort and attention.

FOUNDATIONAL HOME REMEDIES

CHARCOAL POULTICE

Why it's used:
Charcoal has long been valued for its drawing action. Applied externally, it supports clearing and containment at the site of concern.

Basic preparation:
Activated charcoal is mixed with water to form a paste and applied to cloth before placement on the skin.

Use rhythm:
Used in short applications during periods of acute need.

Notes:
External use supports focused, localized care.

primary support areas

bites and stings
skin irritation
localized infection support
foreign matter and splinters

Plant Reference by Support Area

This reference groups plants by the primary areas of support they are traditionally associated with. Many plants appear in more than one section, reflecting the interconnected nature of herbal care.

Digestion & Gut Support
Activated Charcoal, Bitters, Burdock Root, Chicory Root, Dandelion Root, Fennel Seed, Gentian Root, Ginger, Lemon Balm, Licorice Root, Marshmallow Root, Nettle Leaf, Peppermint, Slippery Elm, Triphala, Turmeric

Nerves & Sleep
Ashwagandha, Catnip, Chamomile, Damiana, Lavender, Lemon Balm, Motherwort, Oatstraw, Passionflower, Reishi, St. John's Wort, Tulsi (Holy Basil), Valerian

Hormone & Cyclical Support
Ashwagandha, Black Cohosh, Cramp Bark, Dong Quai, Evening Primrose, Kudzu Root, Maca Root, Motherwort, Mugwort, Red Clover, Red Raspberry Leaf, Vitex (Chasteberry), White Peony, Yarrow

Immune & Respiratory Support
Astragalus, Calendula, Echinacea, Elderberry, Elderflower, Garlic, Ginger, Hibiscus, Licorice Root, Marshmallow Root, Mullein, Oregano, Peppermint, Reishi, Rosemary, Rosehips, Sage Leaf, Schisandra Berries, Spearmint, Thyme, Tulsi (Holy Basil)

Pain & Inflammation Support
Boswellia, Cayenne, Chamomile, Cleavers, Comfrey (Topical), Devil's Claw, Ginger, Skullcap, Turmeric, White Willow Bark

Skin & Lymph Detox
Burdock Root, Calendula, Cayenne, Chickweed, Cleavers, Dandelion Leaf, Echinacea, Ginger, Nettle Leaf, Poke Root, Red Clover, Yellow Dock

Circulation & Heart Support
Cayenne, Garlic, Ginkgo, Ginger, Hawthorn Berry, Hawthorn Leaf & Flower, Hibiscus, Motherwort, Red Sage Root (Danshen), Rosemary, Rose Petals, Schisandra Berries, Turmeric, Yarrow

Energy, Mood & Vitality
Ashwagandha, Eleuthero, Ginger, Kudzu Root, Lemon Balm, Maca Root, Peppermint, Schisandra Berries, Tulsi (Holy Basil), Yerba Mate

Honoring Indigenous Lineages of Plant Knowledge

The plant medicines gathered in this book carry teachings far older than these pages. Across continents and generations, Indigenous peoples have lived in relationship with the land through attentive observation, seasonal rhythm, ceremony, foodways, and collective care. Their knowledge arises from place-based intimacy, lived practice, and responsibility carried over centuries.

Many of the plants referenced here were held, protected, and shared through Indigenous stewardship long before they entered modern herbal traditions. Their uses developed through community, oral transmission, and direct relationship with Earth rather than extraction or ownership. These lineages remind us that healing has always been relational, shaped by reciprocity, restraint, and respect.

As more people turn toward plant medicine in times of uncertainty and change, it becomes essential to acknowledge whose knowledge made this remembering possible. Honoring Indigenous wisdom means recognizing both its endurance and its ongoing presence. These traditions remain alive through Native communities who continue to protect land, language, ceremony, and medicine despite centuries of disruption.

This book is offered with gratitude to the Indigenous guardians of the lands these plants come from and to the wisdom keepers who have preserved their teachings. May our engagement with plant medicine be shaped by humility, care, and responsibility. May food nourish, community strengthen, and compassion guide the way healing unfolds. And may remembrance lead us back into right relationship with Earth and with one another.

Sustainable Practices, Ethical Sourcing, and Foraging

Relationship with plant medicine begins long before preparation or use. It begins with how plants are encountered, gathered, cultivated, and sourced. Sustainable practice supports both the health of the Earth and the integrity of the medicine itself. Care for the body and care for the land arise from the same attention.

Plants thrive within complex ecosystems shaped by soil, water, climate, and community. When these systems are supported, the plants express resilience and vitality. When they are strained, both medicine and landscape suffer. Approaching plant medicine with awareness of origin strengthens the relationship and honors the living systems that make healing possible.

Ethical sourcing invites consideration of how plants reach the hands that work with them. Many herbs are grown, harvested, and prepared by small farms, cooperatives, and Indigenous stewards who carry deep knowledge of land and season. Choosing sources that prioritize ecological health, fair labor, and respectful harvesting supports the continuity of these practices. Labels, certifications, and transparency offer useful guidance, though relationship and reputation often speak most clearly.

Cultivation offers another pathway of connection. Growing even a few medicinal plants at home deepens understanding of their rhythms, needs, and character. Tending soil, observing growth, and harvesting with intention foster appreciation for the time and conditions required for medicine to mature. This intimacy often shapes how plants are later prepared and used.

Foraging carries particular responsibility. It asks for attentiveness to place, plant population, and timing. Ethical foraging begins with correct identification and clear understanding of a plant's growth habits and abundance. Many medicinal plants thrive widely, while others grow slowly or exist within limited ranges. Gathering from abundant populations and leaving enough for regeneration supports ecological balance.

Restraint forms the foundation of respectful foraging. Taking small amounts, harvesting selectively, and returning often to observe rather than gather allow plant communities to remain healthy. Some plants offer medicine through leaves or flowers rather than roots, allowing continued growth. Others benefit from being left untouched entirely. Learning when to harvest and when to refrain strengthens discernment.

Gratitude shapes sustainable relationship. Acknowledging the plant, the land, and the lineage of knowledge that informs use supports reciprocity. Simple gestures of thanks, care for the surrounding area, and mindful presence reinforce the understanding that plants remain living beings rather than resources to extract.

Seasonality offers guidance. Plants express different qualities throughout the year, and aligning harvesting and use with natural cycles supports both potency and balance. Roots often hold strength during dormancy, while leaves and flowers offer medicine during periods of growth. Attention to season supports harmony between human activity and plant life.

This companion encourages thoughtful sourcing and restrained foraging as acts of care rather than obligation. Each choice contributes to a wider pattern of stewardship. When plants are approached with respect, patience, and humility, the relationship remains reciprocal and enduring.

Sustainable practice supports continuity. It ensures that plants remain available for future generations, that ecosystems retain integrity, and that healing traditions remain rooted in relationship rather than consumption. In this way, working with plant medicine becomes both personal care and collective responsibility.

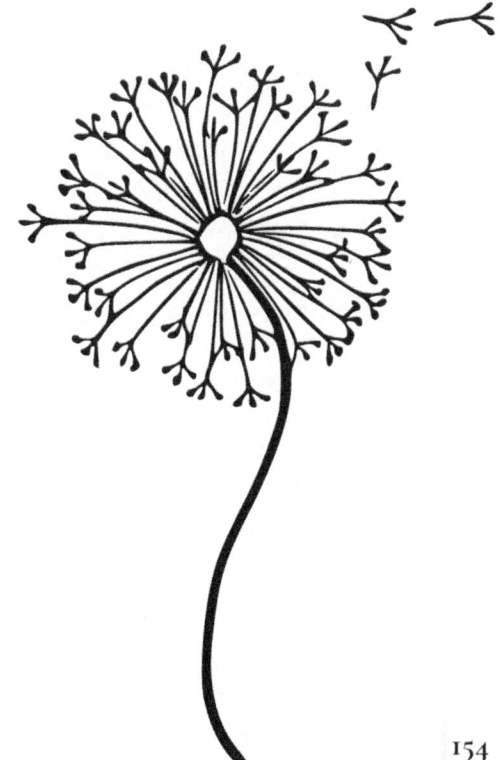

until next time...

As this volume draws to a close, the relationship continues. Every plant gathered with care, every remedy prepared with attention, and every choice made in service of land and community strengthens the living exchange between people and place. Gratitude lives through action here - in tending soil, honoring lineage, and choosing practices that sustain future generations. May the work carried forward from these pages remain rooted in respect, reciprocity, and the quiet understanding that the Earth teaches through continuity as much as through change.

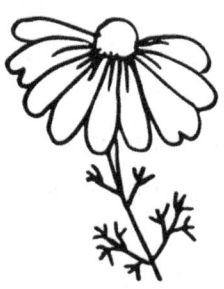

Made in the USA
Coppell, TX
20 January 2026

68446556R00092